AF619204

Dealing with Dementia

Easy To Understand Tips and Resources for Families and Caregivers

© Copyright 2019 - All rights reserved.

The content contained within this book may not be reproduced, duplicated or transmitted without direct written permission from the author or the publisher.

Under no circumstances will any blame or legal responsibility be held against the publisher, or author, for any damages, reparation, or monetary loss due to the information contained within this book. Either directly or indirectly.

Legal Notice:

This book is copyright protected. This book is only for personal use. You cannot amend, distribute, sell, use, quote or paraphrase any part, or the content within this book, without the consent of the author or publisher.

Disclaimer Notice:

Please note the information contained within this document is for educational and entertainment purposes only. All effort has been executed to present accurate, up to date, and reliable, complete information. No warranties of any kind are declared or implied. Readers acknowledge that the author is not engaging in the rendering of legal, financial, medical or professional advice. The content within this book has been derived from various sources. Please consult a licensed professional before attempting any techniques outlined in this book.

By reading this document, the reader agrees that under no circumstances is the author responsible for any losses, direct or indirect, which are incurred as a result of the use of information contained within this document, including, but not limited to, — errors, omissions, or inaccuracies.

Table of Contents

Introduction

You have seen at least one movie where people affected with dementia are depicted more or less accurately. But even with all the widespread coverage of this disease, dementia remains one of the single most misunderstood and least understood diagnoses in the world - both amongst the general population and even in some medical circles.

Most people associate it with psychological issues, but the way dementia develops and the way it affects the life of a person is much different from any psychiatric or psychological problem.

Dementia is a far more complex diagnosis, and understanding it is one of the first steps to make towards dealing with it. Unfortunately, dementia is not fully explained (not all types of dementia, and not entirely) - and, as such, dementia cannot be actually cured, or even treated, per se. Even so, dementia is a medical condition that can be managed through a combination of medical treatments, therapy, and special care. Although these might not be able to treat dementia in the fullest sense of the word, they can make the patient’s life better, and consequently the caretaker's life will be better as well.

Receiving a diagnosis in the dementia spectrum can be extremely shocking both for the person who is receiving the diagnosis and for their loved ones. However, being informed and staying calm in the face of what is to come is extremely important if you want this condition to be managed well.

The book at hand is meant to be an introduction into the world of dementia - an introduction that is not meant to scare you in any way, but help you create a life that is fully adjusted to the difficulties of such a diagnosis.

We will start with an explanation of what dementia actually is and what the main types of dementia are. Contrary to popular belief, Alzheimer’s disease is not the *only* type of dementia. Although similar among their different variations (in most cases), the different types of dementia can have very different onsets and very different evolutions. Knowing where your diagnosis comes from and what it means is essential to managing the disease as well as you can in the years to come, so the chapter addressing this will be the foundation of your knowledge and, hopefully, a good start to help you learn more about what is going on with you (or your loved one).

The chapters following will be dedicated to helping you learn more about the main symptoms of dementia, as well as the main risk factors and the things you can do to reduce the odds of developing such an illness. As you will see in later chapters, dementia can be traced back to a series of medical conditions that are more or less avoidable - but most of the time, the explanation behind its onset is, unfortunately, quite unclear even for the medical corpus.

This is not to say that dementia is completely unavoidable - there *are* things you can do to prevent it and you should definitely do them, especially since they can drastically reduce the odds of developing certain types of more "controllable" types of dementia (such as Vascular Dementia, for example).

Once the basics are established, we will dive deeper into what it means to be diagnosed with dementia. What are the signs that should put you on a doctor's waiting list, and what are the things you should definitely do to make your doctor's visit matter? Even more, what are some of the questions you and your family may have regarding this diagnosis and what is to come after it?

Further on, we will discuss whether or not dementia can be self-diagnosed in any way and if the tests available on the market are of any help in this respect. Hopefully, the answers given in that chapter will help you realize the importance of visiting your doctor as soon as possible.

Last but not least, I will dedicate the largest chapter of this book to describing how to tell friends and family about your diagnosis. You are the only one who can decide when and how (or even *if*) this should be done - but hopefully, the tips offered in that chapter will help you make the right decision. Even more, I hope these tips will help you make sure you break the news as softly as possible - because if there is someone who will be heavily impacted by this diagnosis in the years to come (aside from you, the patient), they will be in your close, immediate family or group of friends.

The latter half of this book will be dedicated entirely to helping you and your family understand what dementia means in terms of changes you will have to bring in your life. Fortunately, as a caretaker, there are many things you can do to make your life easier and to help someone who is suffering from dementia. While this condition might not be curable, it is a condition that can be managed in most cases.

I won't lie: what is ahead of you will not be easy in any way, not as a caretaker and not as a patient. There will be times when things will get so hard you will even ask yourself what you did to deserve this. There will be times of endearment and love, too - because not everything is black when it comes to this type of diagnosis.

I wish you a good, informative reading journey! But more than anything, I wish you strength should a dementia diagnosis be given to you. I hope with all my heart that the book at hand will prove useful in the months and years to come.

Chapter 1: Types of Dementia

Dementia is, perhaps, one of the most misunderstood and one of the least understood diseases in history.

A high-level definition of dementia includes the range of brain diseases that affect the memory, the personality, and the reasoning of a patient diagnosed with this condition.

More often than not, dementia is associated with Alzheimer's - and the association is not entirely wrong, actually. Alzheimer's is, indeed, *one* type of dementia. It is the most commonly known one and one whose symptoms are fairly familiar to a large chunk of the population.

Dementia has been made known to people through a variety of campaigns over the past few years. It would be wrong, however, to assume that just because public awareness has grown recently, research had not been conducted before.

One of the main reasons dementia has grown to be more known in the recent years is related to the growth of the elderly population in general. People live longer than ever before, and natality rates have dropped around the world - therefore, there are more seniors than ever, so the numbers of patients with dementia has also boomed.

In addition to mere numbers, dementia was also made known to the general public by various organizations whose main purpose is that of offering hope to patients and their families. The ardent efforts of these organizations have yielded actual results, not just in terms of making patients and their relatives feel better, but also in terms of engaging governments to provide patients with better care.

The more people were aware of dementia, the more research was funded - and this gave everyone hope. And the more hope there was, the more findings were unveiled. For instance, it was known that acetylcholinesterase inhibitors were tightly connected to Alzheimer's disease, but most researchers did not know that these compounds can alter the pathogenesis of the disease itself. Later on, it was discovered that the same compounds can actually improve memory and cognition in patients.

Although the improvements were not that big, they changed the way people perceived the disease: for the first time, Alzheimer's was not considered an incurable disease anymore, but a treatable one.

New developments are pushed for every day. The road so far is not to be underestimated in any way - but the lack of availability for certain types of treatment and their increased price make them not the best alternative. Therefore, the quest for the best treatment moves on, with research trains focusing on a variety of types of treatment, including treatment based on the patient's genetics and their relation to the onset and development of the disease.

There is hope in the world of dementia research - and that is, perhaps, more important than anything else.

It all starts with a proper understanding of what dementia is - and that it is not only about Alzheimer's disease.

More specifically, here are the main types of dementia:

Vascular Dementia

This disease makes up approximately 10% of the total number of dementia cases, and its onset is connected to the blood vessels that connect the brain. The two main risk factors that lead to Vascular Dementia are the following:

1. Stroke that blocks a brain artery. Although Vascular Dementia is not the only symptom of a stroke, it is a possible one. In many cases, strokes don't even cause noticeable symptoms (but even then, Vascular Dementia is still a risk). Furthermore, the number of strokes one records is directly connected to an increased risk of Vascular Dementia.

2. Chronically damaged or narrowed brain blood vessels. If a patient suffers from a condition that narrows or damages the brain blood vessels long-term, Vascular Dementia becomes a risk. There are multiple conditions that may lead to this, including high blood pressure, aging, atherosclerosis, brain hemorrhage, and even diabetes.

Vascular Dementia does not cause the same degree of memory loss as in the case of Alzheimer's, but sufferers might show trouble organizing, planning, and thinking.

Vascular Dementia does not evolve in a predictable way. Many times, the location as well as the number and size of the brain injuries caused by one or more strokes determine the onset of Vascular Dementia, as well as the degree to which the patient will be affected.

Mixed Dementia

Mixed Dementia occurs when the brain damage has resulted from more than one cause (e.g. both Vascular Dementia-related causes and Parkinson's Disease). Mixed Dementia usually comes on much later in life than other types of dementia and is more likely in patients over 85.

One of the most common examples of how Mixed Dementia develops is when the plaques associated with Alzheimer's Disease are associated with the brain changes of Vascular Dementia.

Dementia with Lewy Bodies (DLB)

Lewy Bodies are clumps of a specific protein that can clog the cerebral cortex, as well as affect the memory and induce thinking problems. More specifically, this type of dementia is connected to alpha-synuclein proteins, which are found in the brain, but whose normal function is not fully known. This type of dementia is frequently characterized by sleeping issues and visual hallucinations.

The symptoms are sometimes similar to those of Parkinson's Disease, but they will vary depending on how the Lewy bodies are moving - sometimes, patients can experience many moments of normality, followed by sudden moments of decline into dementia.

Studies show that Lewy Body Dementia is among the most common types of dementia (following right after Alzheimer's Disease and Vascular Dementia). [1]

The Lewy Bodies underlying this type of Dementia have been found in other brain disorders as well, including Parkinson's and Alzheimer's. Many times, patients with either Lewy Body Dementia or Parkinson's Disease end up experiencing cross-symptoms (e.g. Lewy Body Dementia patients experience body movement issues, while Parkinson's Disease patients experience thinking problems).

Parkinson's Disease

Parkinson's Disease affects the dopamine-producing neurons in a very specific area of the brain. This area of the brain and these neurons are responsible for the movement of

---

[1] Lewy Body Dementia. (2019). Retrieved from https://www.alz.org/alzheimers-dementia/what-is-dementia/types-of-dementia/lewy-body-dementia

the body. The causes of the disease remain largely unknown, but the main symptoms are characterized by problems with movement (slowness, limb rigidity, balance problems, changes in gait and tremor, and so on).

As mentioned before, Parkinson's Disease and Lewy Body Dementia are frequently intertwined, and patients with one of the diseases might experience symptoms of the other disease as well.

Parkinson's Disease is, together with Alzheimer's, among the most well-known types of dementia. One of the most famous examples of a person with Parkinson's Disease was Muhammad Ali, who, after spending his lifetime boxing, developed this disease and lived with it for many years. Michael J. Fox was also diagnosed with Parkinson's at a very young age, but different lifestyle changes and medication have kept him active and working.

Frontotemporal Lobal Degeneration (FTLD)

Frontotemporal Lobal Degeneration is one of the most common types of dementia for people aged under 60 (although there have been cases of FTLD whose onset was recorded as early as 21 and as late as 80)[2]. The disease affects the frontotemporal area of the brain and leads to personality and behavior changes, as well as language difficulties. In most cases, the memory of the patient is well-preserved

In the case of this type of dementia, the nerve cells in the front and the side areas of the brain are especially affected. The progression of the disease varies a lot from one person to another, and it can range between two and twenty years. Furthermore, Frontotemporal Lobal Degeneration can also lead to a general predisposition towards other diseases such as pneumonia, injuries (connected to falling), and infections.

In general, patients diagnosed with FTLD show a life expectancy of seven to thirteen years from the onset of the symptoms. Although there is no cure for this disease, medication and several lifestyle changes can improve the quality of life and even prolong it.

Creutzfeldt-Jakob Disease (CJD)

[2] What is FTD?. (2019). Retrieved from https://www.theaftd.org/what-is-ftd/disease-overview/

This is a very rare brain disorder and it can affect both humans and other mammals. Most often, this disease is referred to as the "mad cow disease" and its onset is popularly connected to eating cow meat from an infected animal. However, the disease can be transmitted through various medical tools that have been used on someone suffering from CJD as well (in 1977, someone was reported to have been infected with Creutzfeldt-Jakob Disease as a result of a brain surgical intervention that used silver electrolytes that had been previously used on a person who suffered from the disease).

Furthermore, aside from acquired CJD, two other categories of this disease must be mentioned: sporadic and familial. Sporadic Creutzfeldt-Jakob Disease appears spontaneously, and it accounts for approximately 85% of the CJD cases.[3] Familial CJD is usually connected to inherited conditions, and it accounts for the majority of the remaining 15% of the total number of CJD cases.

The disease is fatal, and it impairs coordination and memory, affecting behavior as well as the way the brain processes certain types of protein. In most cases, patients pass away within one year from the onset of the symptoms.[4]

About one in a million people in the world are affected by this type of dementia.

Huntington's Disease

This is a progressive brain disorder that is caused by one defective gene or chromosome. Some of the most common symptoms of Huntington's Disease include tremors, jerking, severe decline in thinking and reasoning skills, depression, irritability, as well as a range of other mood changes. As more of the proteins in the brain are affected over time, the disease will get progressively worse.

In most cases, the onset of Huntington's Disease happens in the 30s or 40s, and most patients diagnosed with this disease live fifteen to twenty years. Some very rare forms of Huntington's have a childhood onset. In these cases, the main symptoms are clumsiness, slow movements, rigidity, drooling, and slurred speech. [5]

---

[3] (2019). Retrieved from https://www.who.int/mediacentre/factsheets/fs180/en/

[4] Creutzfeldt-Jakob Disease Fact Sheet | National Institute of Neurological Disorders and Stroke. (2019). Retrieved from https://www.ninds.nih.gov/Disorders/Patient-Caregiver-Education/Fact-Sheets/Creutzfeldt-Jakob-Disease-Fact-Sheet

[5] Reference, G. (2019). Huntington disease. Retrieved from https://ghr.nlm.nih.gov/condition/huntington-disease

Wernicke-Korsakoff Syndrome

Wernicke-Korsakoff Syndrome is a memory disorder that is associated with a severe thiamine deficiency (vitamin B1 deficiency). This syndrome is frequently caused by chronic alcoholism, but this is not the only cause. Most times, symptoms include severe memory problems. Even so, the patient's thinking will most likely seem normal - and once the B1 deficiency is fixed and alcohol consumption is cut back, the patient has a very good chance of restoring the natural balance in the brain.

Wernicke-Korsakoff Syndrome is sometimes associated with Wernicke encephalopathy, a disease that is most often associated with ocular disturbances, off-balance gait and unsteady stance, as well as a general state of confusion.

All of these symptoms are caused by vitamin B1 deficiency as well. This vitamin is an essential coenzyme that is vital in brain functions - so, when it drops, mental changes may occur in a patient. Most of the patients diagnosed with Wernicke encephalopathy are unable to concentrate, become confused, and they may even become unaware of the immediate situations they find themselves in. Moreover, a smaller number of patients may show ocular disturbances (nystagmus) and lateral rectus muscle paralysis. Furthermore, stance problems and gait are among the rarer symptoms, but they should be considered as well if they appear.

In very rare cases, tachycardia, low blood pressure, stupor, hypothermia and loss of hearing can occur as well. Sometimes, patients do not show the main symptoms of the disease, but they experience a selection of the other symptoms - a case in which immediate medical consultation is needed.

Wernicke encephalopathy can be fatal if not treated, leading to coma and death.

As you can see, dementia spans far wider than just Alzheimer's disease alone. Although one of the most common types of dementia and definitely one a large section of the population is familiar with, Alzheimer's is just *one* participant in the entire spectrum of dementia disorders.

Being familiar with all types of dementia is extremely important, because many of them do not show symptoms similar to those of Alzheimer's Disease. Even more, some of them may be commonly connected to each other, and some of them have an early onset as well. The more informed you are, the more you can help yourself and those around you by taking immediate action and visiting a doctor.

In the next chapter, we will go a little more in-depth into the symptoms of dementia and how they are classified, as well as the main causes behind them. My advice is to take this information and internalize it, but always seek the help of medical professional, as this is the only way to get properly diagnosed (and therefore, properly treated as well).

Chapter 2: Symptoms of Dementia

Dementia is not an easy diagnosis, regardless of what type of dementia you or your loved one may have, and regardless of where you stand.

Because this is such a complex range of mental disorders that are frequently interconnected and associated with diseases and medical issues outside of the dementia spectrum, developing a clear diagnosis necessitates a lot of attention and proper investigation.

Even so, being familiar with the high-level symptoms of dementia will help you take action when action is due and visit a doctor for specialized consultation, diagnosis, and treatment.

Many dementia symptoms are common to all the branches of this spectrum of disorders, precisely because they are connected by the definition of dementia itself: a disorder characterized by brain-related symptoms such as memory problems, impaired reasoning, and personality changes.

The symptoms of dementia can be classified in two main categories: the ones related to thinking (cognitive symptoms) and the ones related to the psychology of the individual that has been diagnosed with dementia.

Cognitive changes include the following:

- Memory loss (which is most often noticed by someone close to the patient, rather than the patient himself/ herself)
- Difficulty when it comes to complex tasks
- Difficulty with everyday tasks (e.g. the tasks they would normally run at work)
- Difficulty in communication or in finding the right words to communicate
- Difficulty in situations where reasoning and problem solving capacities are necessary
- Difficulty with coordination and other types of motor functions
- Experiencing moments of confusion and disorientation

Psychological changes can be more subtle at first, so, again, it will most likely take someone else (aside from the patient) to notice them. Very frequently, this category of symptoms include the following:

- Personality changes (a person who might have been quiet will suddenly become louder or more aggressive, and a person who might have been louder will suddenly become more silent)
- Depression and sadness
- Anxiety without an apparent reason
- Developing inappropriate behavior (e.g. being rude, lacking manners, and so on)
- Developing paranoia (e.g. being convinced that someone is spying them)
- Agitation and nervousness (even in situations that are familiar)
- Hallucinations (this is more prevalent in Parkinson's Disease patients)

The Main Causes of Dementia

Although relatively poorly understood (and very commonly *mis*understood), most types of dementia can be traced back to causes that are quite specific. The main cause underlying dementia disorders is the degeneration of the cerebral cortex - the side of the brain that deals with thought processes, memory, personality, and actions. When the brain cells in this side of the brain die, different types of cognitive impairments appear (which is the principal characteristic of dementia in general).

It is extremely important to note that not all causes of dementia are completely incurable. Some of them are treatable. For instance, when dementia is caused by the following problems, it can be treated:

- Head injuries
- Some types of infections (such as HIV/ AIDS, meningitis, and syphilis, which have all been connected to forms of dementia)
- Brain tumors
- Pressure hydrocephalus (characterized by the collection of brain fluids outside of the brain cavities, which pressure it from the exterior)
- Diseases connected to the liver, the kidneys, or the pancreas that affect the

chemical balances of the blood

- Hypoxia (low oxygenation of the blood)
- Nutritional problems (like vitamin deficiencies)
- Drug or substance abuse

Alzheimer's disease, as stated, is the most common type of dementia. Its main cause is an abnormal level of protein deposits in the brain, which leads to degradation of the brain cells in the areas that control mental functions. These proteins (beta amyloids) accumulate when there is an imbalance between the way peptides are produced and then cleared in the body.

The symptoms of Alzheimer's are not easy to notice. In fact, they progress quite a lot before they are noticeable (by the patient or someone close to hem). By the time the symptoms are visible, neuronal loss progress is at high level. Sometimes, it can take up to two decades before a patient starts to experience any of the obvious symptoms.

As was mentioned before, Vascular Dementia is the second most common type of dementia. Atherosclerosis is the main underlying cause for this disorder, which, in turn, is caused by deposits of dead cells, fats, and debris on the insides of the arteries, blocking the blood flow. These blockages can eventually lead to strokes (otherwise explained as interruptions of the blood flow to the brain).

There are several conditions that are frequently associated with atherosclerosis and Vascular Dementia: high cholesterol, high blood pressure, heart diseases, diabetes, and other connected medical conditions. The better these conditions are managed and treated, the lower the odds of developing Vascular Dementia are. If these conditions are discovered and treated after the onset of Vascular Dementia, they might slow down the process of degradation, but once lost, the functions will not be recovered.

What Leads to Memory Loss (Outside of Dementia)

Do keep in mind that just because someone is experiencing one or more of the symptoms of dementia, it does not necessarily mean that they will be diagnosed with it. For instance, memory loss can be caused by a multitude of factors including medication, stress, or sleep deprivation. Furthermore, some of the behavioral changes associated with dementia might also be caused by the aforementioned situations and triggers.

Even so, when one or more symptoms appear, it is of the utmost importance that the patient visits a doctor as soon as possible. Yes, lost functions will not be recovered, but the sooner dementia is managed, the better the quality of the patient's life will be for more time.

If dementia symptoms appear, but a dementia diagnosis is not made, it is important to remove the factors that led to those symptoms. For instance, if memory loss is caused by medication, your doctor can give you similar medication, but without the same side effects.

Alzheimer's Disease Warning Signs

As it was mentioned before, when symptoms of dementia start to be noticeable, the condition is most likely in a fairly advanced state.

However, there are certain warning signs you might want to take into consideration because, as was also mentioned before, the sooner treatment is received, the better it will be for the patient.

With a general aging of the population in the West, being aware of these warning signs becomes even more important, since a lot of people might want to monitor themselves for the development of certain dementia disorders, such as Alzheimer's, for example.

Some of the most common warning signs of Alzheimer's (and other forms of dementia) include the following:

1. The patient may notice a disruption in their daily activities due to memory loss. When this happens, the person might not be able to remember basic things (such as where some of the things in their home are, for example). This leads them to depend on someone else, precisely because they become unable to handle things on their own.

2. The patient may have trouble running simple tasks or planning ahead. For instance, some people might find it hard to manage their finances and their bills, they might find it difficult to follow recipes, and they might take longer to complete very simple tasks.

3. The patient may also find it hard to use tools and technology they did not have trouble using before. For instance, they might temporarily lose their knowledge of how to operate a microwave.

4. The patient may also experience confusion, with occasions when they might not

know what time it is or where they are. In this case, they will easily lose track of hours and days, and they might find themselves in different places without knowing how they got there.

5. Vision problems are also quite common for Alzheimer's patients. A medical specialist can help you determine if the vision issues are connected to Alzheimer's Disease development by running a number of tests.

6. Communication impairment may also develop when someone suffers from Alzheimer's Disease. In these situations, patients will find it difficult to speak or write, they might lose their words, or they might find it unusually difficult to follow conversations (even when they are simple in nature).

7. Patients with Alzheimer's might also develop a tendency to isolate themselves from a social point of view. This is a direct effect of the aforementioned problems, which might make the patient feel like they should be away from the loved ones. However, it is very important to keep in mind that this can actually worsen the condition of the patient.

8. Losing objects is also common with Alzheimer's patients. Frequently misplacing and/or completely losing important things (such as the keys to the house or even money) are two warning signs you should pay attention to.

9. Patients suffering from Alzheimer's Disease, as well as the loved ones around them, might also notice a decreased ability to judge situations or make decisions. For instance, patients might not use their money adequately, or they might give out large sums of money on unnecessary (and even scammy) products.

As a result of poor judgment, patients with Alzheimer's Disease might also stop taking care of themselves (which includes leaving behind basic grooming habits as well).

10. Mood swings are also quite frequent in the case of those who suffer from Alzheimer's. Depression is the most common mood change experienced by these people, but sometimes, other types of behavioral or psychological changes may appear. For instance, the patient may develop anxiety and feel fearful without a concrete reason. Some patients may also become more aggressive.

One of the saddest things about Alzheimer's Disease is that you cannot actually prevent it entirely. There are actions and habits that can help you keep your brain functioning for a long(er) period of time - but even so, the onset of Alzheimer's is frequently connected to factors outside of one's power or control.

While other types of dementia can be avoided up to a certain extent (as you will see in the following chapter), Alzheimer's is so common precisely because there is no underlying cause that can be completely avoided.

Even with all this, the sooner the patient is diagnosed and starts receiving treatment, the slower the disease will progress, allowing those who suffer from Alzheimer's to live happier for a longer period of time.

The next chapter is dedicated to explaining the major risk factors associated with dementia and what you can do to reduce your odds of developing any of the disorders in this spectrum. Taking care of your mind and body can make a difference in a lot of cases, and it can completely change the age at which dementia arises, as well as how fast it progresses in your specific case.

Every person is different, and the development of dementia disorders is different in each and every case. However, following some general, basic rules can help you avoid the worst of the scenarios. So, it is truly important that you are aware of the factors that might reduce risk when it comes to dementia onset and development.

Chapter 3: Risk Factors and How to Reduce Your Risk

Unfortunately, there is no clear recipe on how you can avoid developing a dementia disorder, as sometimes the underlying causes of these conditions are outside of anyone's control.

Research into dementia epidemiology has made considerable advances in the last few years, showing that there might be some level of correlation between dementia disorders and a series of factors, including the location on the globe, genetics, and so on.

One of the most important questions posed by the researchers in this field is whether or not the variations in a gene called APOE 4 are connected to why dementia is more prevalent in some parts of the world or some segments of the global population.

APOE is the short term for Apolipoprotein E gene, a specific type of gene that is responsible for carrying cholesterol in the bloodstream. Research has shown that this gene lies at the fundamental understanding of early-onset dementia, as well as forms of dementia that are associated with genetics. When this gene becomes mutated, the people carrying it will also carry something called a polymorphic allele - and those who carry this E4 allele are at more of a risk of developing dementia.

APOE4 is considered to be a major risk factor not just in the case of dementia disorders, but also in the case of several types of vascular diseases and general cognitive decline that appears with aging (outside of the dementia spectrum).

While the presence of this gene is associated with higher risks, it is important to note that not everyone with this gene will *definitely* develop dementia.

APOE4 seems to have quite the relevant role in the onset and development of dementia, so many scientists are considering treatments that target this gene. This is a plan for the future, though, as no medication has been developed in this direction so far.

What the research done to this moment can help with, however, is determining whether or not you are a carrier of this gene (and thus, pose a higher risk of developing a dementia disorder). Although the information related to this gene is scarce and many medical professionals are skeptical about it, it can still be a fairly good starting point in increasing the measures you take to reduce your risks.

Of course, there are an array of other factors that can influence the onset of dementia, but the example of APOE4 is given here to help you understand that constant research is done in this field and that there is *hope* for the future in many respects.

This hope is largely related to the fact that the population of the world is aging - and thus, Alzheimer's Disease, dementia, and other medical conditions that are usually associated with old age have become a public health concern both in the developed and the developing world. Not only is this a concern from the point of view of the quality of life, but it is a concern from a cost-related point of view, both at the level of the individual and at the level of society as a whole.

There are multiple reasons why governments and non governmental institutions invest a lot of time and financial resources into dementia-related research. Some of the strongest ones include:

1. The fact that dementia is known to shorten the expectancy of life
2. Dementia is a medical condition that deteriorates the cognitive and physical functioning of the patients - and it does so in a progressive way
3. Dementia patients have to be permanently taken care of and monitored
4. Dementia incidences and prevalence are high, and they increase exponentially with the age of the population

Understanding dementia down to its very core is still a challenge for the medical community. This is mostly related to the multitude of factors that lead to the development of dementia disorders and to the way they are sometimes interconnected.

Detecting any kind of risk factor that might help with the prevention and a decrease in occurences of dementia is extremely important, both from the point of view of the individuals diagnosed with the disorder and from the point of view of society in general.

Research until now has uncovered a series of risk factors, most of which are related to Vascular Dementia and have been mentioned above as well: diabetes, atherosclerosis, evidence of ischaemia, alcohol consumption, systolic hypertension at very high levels, high cholesterol and saturated fats in the blood, and so on.

Furthermore, research points to a connection between using diuretics as antihypertensive medication and dementia (patients who take diuretics are less likely to develop dementia).

Of all the medical conditions specific to the elderly, dementia is one of the most common ones. Moreover, it is a common cause of disability and mortality in old age as well. Around the world, more than 50 million people live with dementia. In the United States, 5.7 million people suffer from conditions associated with this spectrum of disorders. These numbers are expected to grow exponentially as the population of the entire world continues aging.[6]

While it is frequently debated *how* common dementia is and to what extent statistics include very mild and mild dementia, one thing is certain: it is a spectrum of disorders that affect the lives of patients and those around them, leading to disability and death.

Understanding the main risk factors behind dementia is, thus, crucial - even more so since anyone can be affected by Alzheimer's, Vascular Dementia, or other types of dementia.

The most common risk factors associated with dementia include the following:

Age

By far, this is one of the most prevalent risk factors of dementia. While cases of Alzheimer's have been reported as early as in the 40s and 50s, dementia is more common with older people. It has been shown that 10% of the population over 65 is suffering from Alzheimer's Disease. Even more, almost one full third of the people aged over 85 suffer from Alzheimer's Disease.[7]

Do keep in mind that, as was mentioned at the beginning of this book, not all forms of dementia are Alzheimer's. Being the most common type of dementia, though, the statistics are more concludent in terms of numerical revealings.

Genetics

We have already touched upon this at the beginning of this chapter. Research shows that the presence of some genes might make the development of dementia more likely to happen. A family history of Alzheimer's also makes it more likely for someone to develop the same disease as well.

At the same time, research shows that a lot of people with a family history of dementia

---

[6] Dementia: Incidence and Prevalence. (2019). Retrieved from https://www.asha.org/PRPSpecificTopic.aspx?folderid=8589935289§ion=Incidence_and_Prevalence

[7] Alzheimer' s Disease Questions and Answers. (2019). Retrieved from https://dshs.texas.gov/alzheimers/qanda.shtm

(Alzheimer's, Creutzfeldt-Jakob disease, Gerstmann-Straussler-Scheinker, and so on) do not suffer from the same afflictions.

Furthermore, it has also been noticed that a lot of people with Down's Syndrome develop signs of Alzheimer's when they reach middle-age as well, making them a group more likely to develop this disease.

Alcohol and Smoking

In general, any kind of substance abuse is bad for your body. However, smoking and the frequent use of alcohol are more commonly associated with dementia. These habits tend to increase the risk that your mental activities decline, they increase the risk of atherosclerosis, and they increase the risk of other vascular diseases (associated with Vascular Dementia in particular).

Regarding alcohol consumption, studies are quite intriguing. On the other hand, large consumption of alcohol is linked to a higher likelihood of dementia. However, drinking moderate amounts of alcohol seems to pose a lesser risk than not drinking at all.

Atherosclerosis

This medical condition is characterized by the buildup of fatty substances, cholesterol, and other debris on the inner lining of your arteries. This buildup is usually referred to as "plaque."

Atherosclerosis is mostly associated with Vascular Dementia (as the artery plaque can block the transport of blood to the brain, which can, in turn, lead to vascular accidents at the brain level).

It is worth noting that some studies also connect atherosclerosis with Alzheimer's Disease as well.

Cholesterol

As it was pointed out above, cholesterol is one of the major, underlying causes for atherosclerosis, which can consequently lead to Vascular Dementia.

However, research shows that there might also be a connection between high levels of cholesterol and Alzheimer's Disease.

Diabetes

Aside from the major health effects diabetes can have on one's life, it is also linked to both Vascular Dementia and Alzheimer's Disease, and one of the main ways it is connected to these conditions is through the high prevalence of diabetes patients who develop atherosclerosis and pose a higher risk of stroke.

Plasma Homocysteine

This blood component is an amino acid whose levels might be affected by a low intake in B6 and B12 vitamins in their diets. A higher level of this amino acid in the blood has been linked with some forms of dementia, including Alzheimer's.

Mild Levels of Cognitive Impairment

Cognitive impairment is not a symptom solely encountered in patients suffering from different forms of dementia. When not connected to dementia, mild cognitive impairment increases the risk that the patient will develop dementia as well. This does not mean that everyone with mild cognitive impairment will suffer from a type of dementia - but it is a risk to be aware of.

Race and Ethnicity

Research has shown that some races and ethnicities are more likely to develop dementia. More specifically, African Americans are more than twice as likely to develop dementia than caucasians, and hispanics are 1.5 times more likely to develop dementia than caucasians.[8] This is not connected to race per se, but to the larger prevalence of cardiovascular diseases among these groups of people (which is also connected to a diet that is usually higher in carbohydrates and fried foods).

Diet

Yes, diet can also play a role in the onset and development of dementia. In general, saturated fats and foods that are generally known to cause cardiovascular diseases should be avoided.

Even more, sugar is a very important dietary ingredient to avoid as well, as its effects have been closely connected with the development of dementia (as well as other diseases not related to this spectrum).

Generally, a diet that is low in carbohydrates and higher in unsaturated fats, lean protein, and vegetables can help you maintain a younger and healthier body. Consequently, this will have a positive impact on the health of your brain as well, protecting you from Alzheimer's Disease and other types of dementia.

Of course, it is not a guarantee that if you eat healthier you will not develop dementia. However, this entire chapter and the tips here are all about preventing the onset of this brain disorder as much as can be done.

Head Injuries

Some forms of dementia begin with physical head injuries. While you may not be able to fully protect yourself from accidents, it is definitely worth noting that you should try to protect yourself as much as possible.

Do keep in mind that not every head trauma resulting in confusion and other symptoms common with dementia will automatically lead to its development.

---

[8] Matthews, K. (2019). Retrieved from https://www.alzheimersanddementia.com/article/S1552-5260(18)33252-7/abstract

Exercise

This is not a risk factor, but something you can do to protect yourself from dementia. Exercising improves blood circulation and helps your brain function better, thus lowering the odds that you will develop any of the disorders in the dementia spectrum.

What is *not* a cause?

For many years, suggestions have been made that connected aluminum in food (e.g. aluminum wrapping) to a higher risk of Alzheimer's. However, even though it's been more than a century since this theory was released for the first time, no study has ever created a plausible bridge between the two.

This is not to say that soda cans and aluminum-wrapped foods are healthy - excess aluminum can still hurt the body in a multitude of ways. However, Alzheimer's has not been proven to be linked with the "consumption" of aluminum through antacids.

These are some of the most common and widely accepted risk factors when it comes to dementia. But what are some of the things you can actively start doing today to protect your body and your brain from developing such an incapacitating disease?

Well, it's all about living a generally balanced life. Alcohol consumption, sugar consumption, a lack of vitamin B1, lack of sleep, lack of physical and mental (yes, mental!) exercise - these can all contribute to the melange of factors that could influence the onset of Alzheimer's Disease or other types of dementia.

The human body is a perfectly built mechanism, with all of its main components and "cogs" working together to keep you alive and feeling well. When one element of this "machinery" breaks, it is frequently likely that it will generate a snowball effect if not treated correctly.

Take care of your body. Be gentle with it. Laugh more, be more social, and train your muscles and your brain in equal measure. These small things can make a difference in the end, offering you a longer, happier life with the ones you love.

Chapter 4: When You Should See Your Doctor

While most types of dementia are not curable or reversible, going to the doctor as soon as the first signs appear is extremely important.

To understand why this is crucial, you should also understand dementia a bit more in-depth. The term comes from Latin, where it was composed out of two words: "de" (which means "separation") and "mens" (which means "mind"). So, if we have to take it in the most literal sense of the word, dementia is about a "separation of the mind" (or a "contraction of the mind" in some translations).

Dementia is not new to mankind. Ancient cultures acknowledged it and even distinguished it from other brain-related conditions, such as delirium. For instance, Aurelius Cornelius Celsus wrote about the distinctions between the two in the first century AD. This is also considered the first time "dementia" was used to describe a medical condition.

Although the distinction lines between the characteristics of dementia and delirium are still somewhat blurred, it is impressive to think that dementia has been debated for literally thousands of years. For instance, some symptoms of delirium are associated with dementia as well. An example of this includes excitement and restlessness. However, both of these symptoms are experienced and perceived in different ways: when it comes to dementia, they refer to agitation and a general disturbance of activities (rather than the frenzy and exaggerated energy experienced by patients with delirium).

No matter which of the dementia disorders you may look at, you will soon understand that these medical conditions are not simple at all. A common cold can be diagnosed and treated at home with hot drinks and bedrest. Dementia, however, cannot and should not be diagnosed by anyone other than a medical professional specialized in this type of disease.

The reason dementia is so complex is because a series of factors have to be taken into consideration when running a diagnosis:

- The history of the onset (when the first symptoms appeared)
- The evolution of the symptoms
- The general medical history of the patient
- A psychiatric evaluation of the patient

- The social and occupational history of the patient
- The family history of the patient
- Comprehensive analysis of the serum electrolytes, urea, liver functions, and glucose
- An analysis of the blood count
- An analysis of B12 vitamin levels, as well as folate values
- An analysis of the thyroid functions
- Neuroimaging evaluations such as a magnetic resonance imaging (MRI), computer tomography (CT) scan of the brain, a single photon emission tomography (SPECT) scan, an electroencephalographic (EEG) test, and so on.
- Genetic and chromosomal tests (important in diagnosing Huntington's Disease and Alzheimer's Disease)

All of these verticals represent large groups of risk factors associated with dementia, as they were presented in the previous chapter.

In addition to the complexity of the tests run to diagnose dementia, it is also important to note that some brain-related conditions may also show the same functional symptoms of dementia. This means that a differential diagnosis will have to be made.

For example, someone who suffers from psychotic schizophrenia may meet all the criteria to be diagnosed with dementia (poor functioning of cognitive abilities, for instance).

Even more, someone suffering from depression may show, at least temporarily, symptoms of dementia as well (e.g. withdrawal from social activities, poor cognitive issues, confusion, forgetfulness, and so on).

In both of these cases (as well as many others), it is absolutely crucial for the patient to be analyzed by a medical professional experienced in dementia (as well as what differentiates it from other mental disorders).

A professional diagnosis made sooner rather than later can have a positive impact on the development of the disorder and the worsening of the patient's condition.

Due to the nature of the medical condition and the fact that it focuses a lot on impaired judgment, the ones who notice the first signs of dementia are frequently not the patients themselves, but their loved ones.

Some of the red flags that should trigger a trip to your doctor include the following:

- Apparently insignificant memory loss (such as not remembering the name of a person the patient knows very well, or the name of a common object they use on a daily basis)
- A general difficulty in following and keeping up with the conversation around them
- Personality and mood changes (as mentioned before, if someone used to be extremely quiet and is now very aggressive and loud, it might be a sign)
- Losing interest in things the patient used to like or do
- Difficulties in completing tasks they normally used to complete (such as tasks at work)
- Difficulty in figuring out what date it is or how the patient got to some place
- Difficulty following TV shows and/or movies that they have watched before
- Getting lost even in those areas that are fairly familiar

Sometimes, the patient may not be aware that they are having these issues, precisely because that is the nature of these symptoms.

If this is the case and you notice any (or a combination of) symptoms in someone you love, it is crucial to take them to a medical consult as soon as possible.

You might not want to bring up dementia from the very beginning. Instead, you can apply the following tactics:

- Suggest an annual checkup
- Use other physical medical issues as a pretext to visit the doctor
- Talk to the person when they seem more lucid and bring up the issue
- Do not argue with the person. Their entire view on life and judgment is impaired, so it is quite likely that if the disease has progressed it will affect the way the discussion is going

It is highly recommended that someone close to the patient go with them for the first rounds of examinations (and for the following ones as well). This is extremely important, because the patient may not fully remember what the doctor says, the examination appointments, or what they need to do next.

The testing to diagnose any of the dementia disorders will most likely include visits to multiple specialists:

- A neurologist who can determine if the structure of the brain is intact or, if this is not the case, to what degree it has been affected.
- A psychiatrist to determine if certain behavioral changes are a sign of dementia or another disorder (e.g. a mood disorder)
- A geriatrician who specializes in the medical conditions common to older people. This specialist will formulate and prescribe adequate treatment based on the results of the tests and examinations.

Aside from the medical examinations, each of these medical specialists will also test the patient in written form, asking them to perform some tasks or answer some questions. Based on the results from these tests, the doctor(s) will be able to determine if the patient suffers from dementia or not.

Realizing that someone you love might be suffering from a disorder connected to dementia is a difficult milestone. So, to make sure that you will be able to provide them with the help they need, make sure you strengthen yourself.

The following chapters are dedicated to what happens past the point where you realize a doctor's visit is necessary - the moments before you visit the doctor and the moments after the visit and diagnosis. These chapters are meant to be an aid for both patients who have come to the realization of their symptoms on their own and for their loved ones who will stand by their side throughout this journey.

Chapter 5: Make Your Doctor's Visit Count

Once you have decided to visit the doctor and get yourself tested for the various types of dementia, it is extremely important to make the most out of this visit. Sometimes, the time for each visit like this can be quite short, so you should do everything in your power to make sure that it all makes a difference, that you can be diagnosed correctly, and that you remember the explanations given by the doctor.

Here are some of the things you can do before and during your doctor's visit:

1. Keeping a journal with all the symptoms you have noticed about yourself or about your loved one. Do make sure to include:

    - Physical symptoms
    - Memory loss and other mental symptoms that affect your capacity and ability to work or perform daily tasks as you would normally do them
    - Behavioral changes (what they are characterized by, what happened to trigger that change and what happened afterwards, how long the episode lasted, and so on).
    - Notes of the most important milestones (when you noticed the symptoms the first time, if they get worse under certain situations or at certain times of the day, whether or not there are any kind of triggers, such as lack of sleep, stress, new medication, and so on).
    - If the symptoms have changed over time and how
    - Whether or not you tried to do something to improve the memory loss (such as doing brain exercises of any kind, for example).

2. Create a list of all the medication you are taking at the moment. You should include both prescription drugs and over the counter drugs such as vitamins, dietary supplements, herbal remedies, homeopathic remedies, and so on. Furthermore, you should include patches you may be using (such as those that help you stop smoking or those for pain, for example), eyedrops, antacids, and any other medical product you may be "consuming."

Your list should include as much detail as possible: the name of the drug, the dosage (e.g. 25 milligrams), the frequency of the administration (twice a day, for example), the doctor who prescribed it, the reason it was prescribed, how long you have taken it, and any kind of side effects you may have spotted.

If you don't remember these points exactly, the frequency and dosage of the medication is written on the bottle of the prescription drugs. If you are taking non-prescription drugs, bring them to your doctor's visit as well.

Also, it is quite important to remember who prescribed the medicine and why. As we get older, we tend to visit more than one medical specialists, and each of them might have their own recommendation. However, sometimes, the recommendations and medication prescribed by the different doctors can be contradictory or can interact with each other.

Furthermore, you should also consider the main reason you are taking a particular type of medicine. Are you treating a long-term condition (a chronic one) or a short-term, acute one? If it's the second option, you probably don't have to take long-term medication (like opioid pain relievers, for example).

Some types of medication and even some types of over the counter remedies (antacids, for example) have been shown to affect the memory, so it is important to discuss with your doctor whether or not you can remove or replace those with better alternatives.

Because a lot of people in their 50s take multiple types of medication and vitamins every day, there is an ongoing trend in medicine to take people off medication they have been taking for years. However, this should only be done when a doctor prescribes it, because you want to make sure you do not have to continue taking them. Also, you have to make sure that any potential medication replacement will not affect your allergies (e.g. penicillin).

3. Bring pen and paper to take notes. You want to make the most out of every single thing you discuss with your doctor - and you want to make sure you remember it all afterwards as well. Therefore, it is definitely a good idea to bring something you can take notes on - a notebook and a pen will do the trick. Write down all the results of your blood work and cognitive tests, as well as any kind of follow-up steps you should make from here on.

4. Bring someone with you. This is quite important both from the point of view of the support you need in these times and from the point of view of making sure that all of the details you will discuss with your doctor will be remembered and taken note of.

Last, but definitely not least, it is quite important that you go to your doctor with your heart open and with a prepared mindset. Dementia is a hard diagnosis - but keeping yourself optimistic will also help you maintain your state of health for longer.

There are 10 million new cases of dementia recorded every year around the world. More than 60-70% of these cases are Alzheimer's Disease.[9] An early medical investigation will help you get treatment as early as possible and stagnate the evolution of the disease - so it is crucial that you do not postpone this.

As a patient, you will need the support of those who love you. As a person who loves a patient diagnosed with dementia, you will need to be prepared to offer your support and love. A dementia diagnosis can come as a storm in your life, but being strong and staying as positive as possible will definitely help.

The following chapters are all about going in-depth with the types of tests you will have to go through to find a diagnosis, as well as what happens after the diagnosis is set: the questions you may have, how to tell your family about this diagnosis, and how to care for someone who suffers from dementia if your loved one has been diagnosed as such.

[9] https://www.who.int/news-room/fact-sheets/detail/dementia

Chapter 6: Questions about Your Dementia Diagnosis

Being diagnosed with dementia can attract a lot of questions - both from the patient and from those around them.

Probably the most common question is *why* - but unfortunately, that is not a question that can be answered easily in most situations, precisely because dementia is influenced by so many risk factors and situations that there cannot be (and will probably never be) a simple answer.

In fact, dementia is so complex that the medical world is split when it comes to its very nature. Some call it a disorder, while others call it a syndrome. These two terms are highly different in nature because one implies that the connection between the symptoms and the causes is much tighter than in the case of the second. More specifically, a disorder is defined to be a medical condition directly influenced by a physical problem (a disruption in the structure and functions of the body). On the other hand, a syndrome is defined as a medical condition characterized by a collection of symptoms that are associated with a health-related cause.

The distinction is important to understand because it shows just how complex the views on the nature of dementia are, and how complex the research behind it is as well. Even more, understanding this distinction from the point of the medical community may establish a path to a cure (or at least a form of treatment that is more efficient than what we currently have).

If even the medical community itself has questions connected to dementia, it is only natural that *you* have them too, regardless of whether you are a patient or someone close to a patient.

The questions you will have are, most likely, more pragmatic in nature than those of the research, and they will boil down to the essentials you need to understand to proceed further and manage your (or your loved one's) condition as well as you can.

Following, you will find some of the most common questions patient and their dear ones ask when they are diagnosed with dementia, or when they are suspect of this medical condition.

1. What is dementia?

Most often, dementia is defined as a blanket term for a series of medical conditions affecting memory, the ability to think, and the ability to reason. As we have presented it in this book as well, the symptoms of dementia can vary a lot from one person to another, and they can inter-mingle as well. However, most of the time, the high-level definition offers a relatively good explanation of what the patient and their loved ones should expect from the evolution of the medical condition.

2. Is all memory loss defined as dementia?

No. Dementia is an umbrella term used to describe a wider range of medical conditions unified by a series of common symptoms, one of which is memory loss. However, there are many other reasons a person might lose their memory - temporarily or not. Lack of sleep, stress, and certain types of medication are among the most common reasons (outside of the dementia spectrum).

3. Is dementia synonymous with Alzheimer's Disease?

No, it isn't. "Dementia" describes a series of medical conditions differentiated in symptomatology, epidemiology, and causes. In other words, many medical conditions can be defined as "dementia," and Alzheimer's Disease is one of them. Because it is also the most common diagnosis, a lot of people directly juxtapose the two terms. However, other forms of dementia exist, including Vascular Dementia, Huntington's Disease, Parkinson's Disease, and so on.

4. Can Alzheimer's Disease be 100% confirmed as a diagnosis while the person is alive?

Unfortunately, no. As you will see in our next chapter, where we go in-depth with the diagnosis process behind dementia, there are a series of tests and examinations medical professionals can run to bring them very *close* to a diagnosis of Alzheimer's Disease. However, only autopsy and the examination of the brain tissue can determine with absolute certainty that a person suffered from Alzheimer's Disease.

Other forms of dementia might be easier to diagnose, depending on the exact symptoms and the typology they fall under. However, even with all this, it is important to note that a close diagnosis can actually be enough to provide you with help. The sooner you start making steps to ameliorate your situation, the better you will be able to cope with it in the future.

5. What are the next steps, following a diagnosis?

There is no exact recipe on what to do to "get rid" of dementia. In most cases (except those that have been caused by very physical situations that can be ameliorated), memory loss is not a process that can be reversed. Its progress can be slowed down, though, which can considerably improve one's quality of life.

The first step to take once you or someone you love have been diagnosed with dementia is to read as much as you can about your specific type of diagnosis. This can make a very big difference because it will help you understand why some things are happening and why it is important to follow your doctor's prescribed treatment and recommendations.

The second step is to let the people in your life know about your diagnosis. Isolating yourself from the ones you love and society can lead to nothing good, particularly because dementia is the kind of diagnosis that will require everyone's support. Breaking down the news can be difficult, but it is a crucial step you should not skip - your loved ones *need* and *deserve* to know what you are going through.

The third step is to learn more about the treatments recommended by your doctor and to follow them thoroughly and regularly. While the treatments currently available may not be able to cure or revert the brain degradation process, they can improve your life onwards and help you manage this condition as well as possible.

Furthermore, it is recommended to ask about support groups in your area. Alzheimer's Disease has gained quite a lot of mainstream awareness in recent years, so it is likely that you will find a support group near you. This will help you manage your future better, as having an entire group of people around you who know exactly what you are going through can definitely improve your outlook on this diagnosis.

The fourth step is to start planning your life from hereon. Changes will occur, and it is of the utmost importance that you take them as they are, because it is the safest thing to do, both for you and for your family and loved ones.

Some of these changes may imply:

- Defining your care and who will make the healthcare decisions if you are not able to do it. Do call for the help of a living will or lasting power of attorney, as these documents can help you design a legal plan of action in the eventuality that you will not be able to make decisions for yourself in the future.

- Defining who will administer your finances from hereon. Since memory loss and poor judgment are almost always part of the dementia diagnosis, having someone to manage your finances is the safest thing you can do. You don't have to give over your entire financial management to someone else, but you do need to design a plan in case you stop being able to manage your own financial situation.

- Define what will happen with your dependents. If you have children, grandchildren, or pets, it is important to plan ahead what happens to them if you stop being able to care for them. Furthermore, it is also recommended that you appoint a legal guardian to ensure that you will continue to be taken care of, no matter what.

Some of these plans might involve paperwork, because the documents you leave must be legally admissible in case anything happens and your situation deteriorates. These documents have to be created as soon as possible, because they will only be valid as long as the person behind them (the patient) is able to execute them.

For instance, you might have to design a living trust using the help of an attorney specializing in elder law. The trust could include any of the following:

- Property
- A property plan disposition
- How the trust will be followed should the patient decease

Furthermore, creating a will now is important as well, precisely because creating it at any point further on when your medical situation may get worse might invalidate the document.

Last, but not least, a Durable Power of Attorney for Healthcare and a Do Not Resuscitate Order should be on your list as well. The first one will legally designate the person who takes care of you, while the second one is an optional document you might want to sign if you do not want to be resuscitated.

6. What treatments are available for dementia?

The types of treatments available for dementia depend on the exact form of dementia you have been diagnosed with. Most of the time, though, the medication will be administered to handle the different symptoms you are suffering from. Furthermore, lifestyle changes might be suggested as well. For instance, you might have to exercise more, as this has been connected with a slower cognitive decline even in patients who suffer from Alzheimer's.

Some of the medication you will be given may be effective in varying degrees. Other medications can cause side effects. In most of the cases, the medication may show unwanted side effects. However, it is crucial that you discuss your options with your doctor and find the best treatment for your particular situation.

7. How to cope with memory loss?

As mentioned before, memory loss is not a process that can be undone. However, proper medication and lifestyle changes can help you cope with this condition a little better than otherwise.

There are a series of techniques you can employ to better manage memory loss as well. Here are a couple of examples:

- Label your cupboard doors in the kitchen using labels or sticky notes. This will help you find things easier around your kitchen without having to search through everything. You can do the same with your clothing drawers as well.

- Get a journal or a diary and always jot down all of your appointments and the important information you don't want to forget.

- Get a pill carrier. This will help you make sure you take your medication every time, on time. Since you can take the little boxes out of the big organizer and carry them around, and since the entire organizer is meant to help you keep track of your medication, this is a step you should be sure to make.

- Create routines for everything in your life, from taking off your clothes to putting them in the laundry, from creating shopping lists to running daily tasks. Routines help you stay on track with everything you do, and they lower the odds that you will forget to do something important.

While dementia is not curable, it can be manageable. With the right support system, the correct medication, and a generally positive mindset, you can continue to live a normal and happy life for many years. Yes, you should be prepared for the worst (and this is why you should make sure you have your paperwork and legal documents in order). But you should not necessarily *think* of the worst every second of your life.

Chapter 7: Testing Yourself to See If You Have Dementia

Running a diagnosis on dementia is not an easy task. As explained in previous chapters, dementia is characterized by a long list of symptoms - some of which are common among the different types of dementia, and others are common to other medical conditions as well.

No single test can determine if a person has dementia - and this includes Alzheimer's Disease as well, as the most common and probably the most widely researched branch of the dementia spectrum.

When a person is suspected to suffer from dementia, the doctor will assess all possible causes to determine if that person actually suffers from any of the medical conditions in the dementia spectrum. The first medical professional you will have to visit is your physician, as they are the most familiar with your history and they can make further recommendations based on initial tests.

Most often, the assessment for dementia includes the following stages of testing and examinations:

Assessing the Medical History of the Patient

There are multiple underlying conditions as well as genetic features that might influence whether or not someone develops Alzheimer's Disease or a medical condition associated with dementia.

Some of the most common questions and examinations in this sense include:

- Finding out whether dementia cases have been recorded in the family
- Finding out when and how the main symptoms appeared
- Finding out if the person is taking medication that might cause the symptoms (or even worsen them)
- Finding out if there have been behavioral and personality changes recorded

- Measuring the blood pressure and the basic vital signs (which will help the doctor determine if the patient is suffering from underlying conditions that might cause dementia or might be classified as symptoms of it). Some of these conditions may also be treatable, meaning that improving them might improve the state of the patient as well.

- Running neurological tests. These tests will determine if the patient experiences issues in terms of balance, reflexes, sensory response, or any other cognitive functions. Any of these conditions could potentially affect the diagnosis, and some of them are treatable with medication as well.

To determine all of the above, the patient will most likely have to undergo a series of procedures meant to determine if they are experiencing symptoms of dementia, what type of dementia they may be suffering from, or if their symptoms are not necessarily connected to dementia in general.

Some of the most widely used procedures in these situations include the following:

- Neuropsychological tests and cognitive tests. These examinations are meant to assess the patient's memory, their problem solving skills, their math skills, their language skills, as well as other mental functioning-related abilities.

- Laboratory tests. The patient may have to get their blood and other fluids tested, as this will help them determine if some of the chemicals, hormones, and vitamins in their bodies are at normal levels. This will help the medical professional discover if some symptoms are connected to a dementia diagnosis, or if they can be ruled out.

As mentioned before, memory problems can be caused by a series of issues including kidney problems, anemia, infections, diabetes, liver disease, some types of vitamin deficiencies, issues with the thyroid, cardiovascular problems, or high blood pressure.

- Brain scans. Most of the times, these tests are used to identify if the symptoms experienced by the patient are connected to any form of stroke, tumor, or any other medical condition at brain level that might cause dementia. These tests will also help the doctor determine if there are changes in the structure of the brain and the way it functions. Most often, these brain scans include (but are not necessarily limited to):

    - CT (Computer Tomography) - a scan that uses x-rays to show images of the brain (or other organs)

    - MRI (Magnetic Resonance Imaging) - a scan that uses magnetic fields, as well as radio waves, to create detailed images of different body structures

(such as the nerves, muscles, bones, and so on)

  - PET (Positron Emission Tomography) - a scan that uses radiation to create images of the brain activity

- Psychiatric evaluations. This will help your doctor determine if the symptoms you are experiencing are caused by other types of mental health conditions (aside from dementia). For instance, depression can cause confusion and forgetfulness, but it is not considered to pertain to the spectrum of medical conditions generally referred to as "dementia."

- Genetic tests. As was explained earlier in this book, some genes may influence whether or not someone develops dementia. Combined with other examinations and tests, this can lead to a more accurate diagnosis. Even more, some types of dementia are directly connected to genetic issues. For instance, Vascular Dementia may be related to genetic heritage, and some studies have shown that Lewy Bodies Dementia might be connected to certain traits of the genetic structure as well.

So, who diagnoses dementia?

Most often, visiting your physician/ family doctor will be the first step. As the examinations progress, your family doctor may also recommend you visit other specialists - psychiatrists, neuropsychologists, geriatricians, and so on.

Some communities may not have a dementia specialist in the vicinity. In these cases, you can address the neurology department of the local hospital or medical school, as they can refer you to someone who can help.

Home Screening Tests for Dementia

The market is full of home screening tests for dementia. While they might provide you with a fairly accurate view on *some* aspects connected to dementia, they should never replace a full consultation done by a medical professional. As was shown throughout this book, dementia is far too complex to be diagnosable by running a few simple tests at home.

Most of these home screenings test a person's cognitive abilities, such as:

- Testing the mental status - the memory, the ability to solve simple problems, other cognitive skills (remembering words, doing math calculations, and so on)

- Testing whether the person can locate themselves in time and space
- Mini-mental state exams (MMSE). These tests are usually used by medical professionals to determine the mental skills of patients. Some of these tests are available online as well, and they allow those who test themselves to identify signs of dementia in general or Alzheimer's in particular. In the latter case, it has been noticed that general scores for these screenings go down a few points every year, showing that the cognitive skills are declining.
- Mini-cog tests (or mini-cognitive tests) will require you to complete two tasks: remember and then a few minutes later repeat the names of three usual objects and draw a face of a clock showing a specific time mentioned by the examiner.
- SAGE tests (self-administered gerocognitive exam), which are designed to detect the earlier signs of cognitive, memory, or thinking problems.
- FDA-approved computerized tests. Some companies have created and marketed cognitive tests available for the wide population. The Automated Neuropsychological Assessment Metrics (ANAM) is one of the most important and popular devices in this category. The tests on this device have been developed with the help of the military, and most of the time, they are used by doctors to assess a patient's likelihood to be diagnosed with dementia. However, some of these tests are also available online for home screenings.
- Neurotrack tests track the cognitive function of a person over time to detect the specific degree of decline. This test is paid and it costs $99, but it might be covered by different health insurance policies as well.
- Memtrax tests, which are also meant to test cognitive functions. This type of test is available for free online.

All of these tests can prove helpful in determining whether or not you are showing signs of dementia. However, they should *never* replace an actual diagnosis made by a team of medical professionals.

Yes, these tests can be revealing in spotting if you have symptoms that are generally associated with dementia. However, and this must be emphasized, not all of these symptoms are *always* associated with dementia. Sometimes, the underlying cause of memory loss, confusion, or loss of cognitive abilities might be connected to anything *but* dementia - and only proper medical examinations and professionals can determine if that is the case.

Chapter 8: Telling Family and Friends that You Have Dementia

Aside from finding out that you suffer from dementia, one of the most difficult moments of this journey will be telling your family and friends about it.

No matter how hard it may be, though, it is important that you do it. You need all of their love and support in this, and they deserve to know so that they can mentally prepare themselves for the situations they might have to face in the future.

In the end, it is entirely your choice if you choose to inform those close to you about your condition. It is understandable that, under certain circumstances, you may not want to reveal this information to those around you - and it is a decision everyone should respect from every point of view.

There are a few reasons you should think long and hard before you decide not to tell them, though. One of the most important ones is connected to the fact that these people *love you* and they really want to provide you with all the support you need.

The second reason is related to the fact that, if the medical condition progresses, you might be in danger (and you might pose a danger to those around you as well). Nobody likes to think of the worst case scenarios, but being prepared is always better than being taken by surprise in these situations. Therefore, it would probably be best for your family and friends to know about your condition and to be prepared themselves for the moments to come.

What are some of the things you should do before you tell your family and friends about being diagnosed with dementia - and how do you actually do it?

This chapter is all about that: letting those you love know that you are suffering from dementia and making sure that the news will be broken in as smoothly as it can be. Nobody can take this kind of news lightly - but doing some things before you break the news can actually help a lot.

Criteria to Consider When Breaking the News

First, Educate Yourself

Your family and friends will most likely have plenty of questions. *You* did when you first learned about the diagnosis, so it's only natural that they do, too. In order to be able to answer their immediate questions, it is important to educate yourself first and foremost.

Fortunately, there are a lot of resources that can help you understand dementia and what you are about to go through. Read everything, ask questions, and be prepared to break the news to your family knowing as much as possible.

For instance, every type of dementia has its own prognosis, so if your family and friends are more familiar with Alzheimer's Disease, but you are diagnosed with a different type of dementia, they might think of a certain outcome for your condition. Knowing how and what to explain to them will help them understand the situation better.

Furthermore, you can also give your family and friends brochures and website links to help you convey the message you want to share with them. It may not be a message about the actual medical condition itself, but a message about what they should expect in the following years, and what you hope they will be able to help with.

Consider Your Age

When deciding how to break the news to your closest ones, consider your age. The higher the number, the more different the outlook of dementia will be. Furthermore, if you are in your 80s, breaking the news to your loved ones might be easier, as it might not come as shocking for your family. Unfortunately, dementia can come on as early as the 40s and 50s - cases in which it is quite important that you are even more careful with how you inform your loved ones.

Marital Status

If you are in a stable relationship or if you are married, you should consider this as well. A diagnosis of dementia can put a real strain on a relationship, and it can make the patient feel like he/she is a burden to their partner.

For both of the people involved in the relationship, the diagnosis can be terribly frightening, precisely because the future becomes more unpredictable than ever. Every person responds differently to every type of dementia. There are treatments available for Alzheimer's Disease and other forms of dementia, and new advances are made every day. However, the future is still uncertain for those bearing with them such a diagnosis and for those who are closest to them.

Your spouse or your life partner should be aware of the situation in the fullest sense of the word. It might be difficult to tell them this, but it is the healthiest thing you can do - for you and for them.

Deciding Who You Should Tell

You don't have to tell everyone in your life that you suffer from dementia. You don't *have to* tell anyone if that is your choice (but do keep in mind that this will attract consequences you should be aware of when you make this decision).

If you decide to tell a few people in your life about your diagnosis, it should be the people you are close to. Decide how important it is for you that they know about this.

Another aspect you should keep in mind is how broken the person will be when hearing about the news. If you think the other person could not take the news and that it would devastate them, consider if you should tell them or not.

Last, but not least, consider how likely it is for a person to remain in your life after knowing the news and how likely it is that they will offer you the physical and practical support as time goes by.

Dealing with Alzheimer's and integrating it in your life is not easy at all. But sharing the news with your loved ones can help you *a lot*, and it can help them be prepared for what is to come as well. It is understandable why you might not want to share the news with everyone or even with certain people, given that you might be thinking that this diagnosis will have an impact on how those people perceive you. However, an Alzheimer's Disease or dementia diagnosis is not your fault. Those who love you will understand this, and they will stand by you no matter what.

In the end, it is important to be comfortable with the people you want to break the news to. Start small by only telling your very inner circle of friends and family about it. You can always tell more people later on if needed, or if you feel that it would be beneficial. The most important thing right now is that you feel supported by those you love the most.

Choose the Right Moment and Manner

Informing those you love that you have been diagnosed with dementia is your choice in every respect - including the moment and the way you choose to do it. It is important to consider all of the aforementioned criteria and to construct your message in a way that makes the news as soft as it can be given the situation.

Some patients choose to break the news to their friends and family in one on one discussions. Other patients, however, choose to do this by organizing a gathering and telling everyone at the same time, as well as answering any immediate questions the people might have when hearing the diagnosis.

When you tell the news, the person in front of you (or the group of people) should be relaxed and not too agitated, as the information may come as more of a shock otherwise. Also, you should make your message as clear as possible, so writing down what you want to say might help (this might also help you come to terms with how you will define "normal" from hereon).

Further Information on What's Next

As mentioned before, every patient experiences dementia differently. Therefore, you cannot fully prepare yourself or those around you on what comes next and how you will react to the medical condition as it progresses.

What you can do, however, is provide them with information on what can be done to make the progress slower, on the therapies available, as well as on the lifestyle changes you might have to make to adjust to your diagnosis.

Therapies Associated with Dementia

In recent decades, dementia and Alzheimer's Disease have grown to be much better known by the general public. These medical conditions may not always be understood, but most people are familiar with what they imply, at least at a very general level.

What people who have not had to deal with dementia may not know, however, is that treatments and therapies are much more widely available today than a few decades ago. While neither medical treatment nor therapies can actually *cure* dementia, they can improve the life expectancy and, overall, the life quality of both the person diagnosed with dementia and those around them.

Following, we will make an introduction into some of the most widespread therapies associated with dementia management. Of course, you should discuss these with your doctor, and they by no means replace conventional medication, but knowing about them (and informing your loved ones about them) might help you build a better outcome for your diagnosis.

Reality Orientation Therapy

Reality orientation therapy was developed as a structured program at the end of the 1950s in the U.S., and are now used at a worldwide level.

This therapy was not initially developed for patients with dementia or Alzheimer's, but for people who were disoriented and/or neglected. However, therapists these days are using it with people suffering from dementia as well, and the results are quite promising.

There are three main components of this therapy:

- 24-hour process, which happens continuously throughout a day and which implies that the patient is constantly reminded of every interaction, the time, the place, the people, and the events happening around them. The person helping the patient should also answer any questions he/she might have.
- Sometimes, reality orientation classes are given daily for about 30-60 minutes. These classes involve patient(s) repeating simple pieces of information such as the date, the weather outside, the names of the people around them, and so on.
- Attitude therapy is applied by the people around the patient (staff, family, friends). In this component of reality orientation therapy, the people surrounding the patient will chose one of a number of attitudes to use with the patient. This way, everyone will be behaving with the patient the same way, eliminating the odds of confusion.

Reality orientation therapy might sometimes involve environmental changes as well, such as the use of memory aids or signs, for example. These aids point the patient to the place where they can find answers to some of their most common questions. This enables the patient to be as self-sufficient as possible, which also improves their mood and helps them feel better about their situation.

This therapy is frequently used in combination with other types of therapies (some of which will be described further on in this book as well). Throughout all of these practices, however, one element dominates: a positive attitude. Communication with the patient always involves listening as much as talking, and respect is always there.

While it may not be able to reverse or eliminate dementia symptoms (as nothing does), reality orientation therapy can help patients feel more anchored in the surrounding, immediate reality of their lives. This therapy focuses a lot on boosting the patient's morale by constantly training them to handle themselves on their own for a wide range of situation. Therefore, the therapy can be considered to be meaningful and helpful for both patients and the ones around them.

Reminiscence

This is not a therapy, per se, but a technique that can help patients suffering from dementia.

Some might be afraid that it will distress the patient to talk about the past when one of their main symptoms is forgetfulness. However, in most cases, people suffering from dementia can easily recall the distant past, while they find it very difficult to recall far more recent events. Therefore, they will find it easier to talk about what happened in the past, rather than talk about what is happening in the here and now.

Reminiscence can take a few shapes when dealing with dementia patients. It can be a life review, a recall of their life history, a story in the patient's life, or a simple reminiscence.

This therapy is still being researched, and there are no conclusive results on how exactly it works. However, the main theory is that it helps patients stay as far from despair as one possibly can.

For instance, life review reminiscence therapy is used in the last phase of life, and its main goal is acceptance. This type of therapy should only be applied with the patient's consent and it should **only be performed by trained therapists**.

On the other hand, simple reminiscence has an easier goal: that of helping the patient communicate, socialize, and remember nice moments. This form of therapy can be either individual or group-based, it can be structured or not, it can be spontaneous or not, and it can be very general or very specific. This therapy should also be performed by **trained** therapists, because sad memories might emerge - and in those cases, the patient needs someone experienced to handle this kind of situation.

It is important for you to also understand that there is a difference between life story therapy and life history therapy. While the latter is all about sharing a person's story (often within group therapy sessions), the first is more complex because it includes certain current aspects of the patient's life. The main purpose behind it is to allow the people present, as well as the patient themselves, to see beyond the illness.

Furthermore, life story therapies can also help the patient make sense of their past and present and connect the dots between the two. Often, this therapy is employed using different types of materials, such as photos, written information, videos, newspaper cuttings, and so on.

Again, and this must be emphasized, reminiscing should only be practiced under the close supervision of someone who is actually experienced in managing this type of therapy in the event that things go wrong.

Validation Therapy

Also developed in the U.S., validation therapy focuses on communicating with elderly people who are disoriented. The main idea behind this therapy is offering these patients validation and support for their feelings, regardless of where the patients may think they are or if they know the time they finds themselves in.

For instance, patients diagnosed with dementia may talk about people in their lives who have passed away as if they were still alive. In validation therapy, the therapist sees this as a need, rather than a simple confusion. More specifically, therapists see this as a need for something the person who is not alive anymore offered to the patients (e.g. parents offer protection, so when patients talk about their parents as if they are still alive, they are in need of protection).

In these cases, confronting the patient with the reality might make them feel too sad and it might make them withdraw from the moment. Sometimes, they might even become hostile.

The main purpose behind this therapy is to make the patients feel dignified and to prevent them from withdrawing into themselves. An empathic listener that does not judge and accepts the patient's momentary reality will help them deal with past moments that might be painful, or simply to provide them with closure for past situations in their lives.

It is important to mention that this therapy is also employed by trained specialists, precisely because it might trigger very bad moments for the patient. Furthermore, there are techniques specific to this therapy that should only be used by professionals in the field.

Dealing with Behavior Modification

Behavior problems are common in multiple types of dementia, and a lot of patients end up experiencing symptoms in this area.

Therefore, behavioral therapies are sometimes employed by therapists dealing with dementia patients. More specifically, these approaches are used when working with patients that experience wandering, aggression, or screaming.

The behavioral tactics can be used to help the learning process when learning is still possible for the patient who suffers from dementia. This approach can help the learning process by creating the environmental conditions for new behaviors to be learned (or older behaviors to be maintained).

Research on the efficiency of this type of therapy can be contradictory at times. On the one hand, some studies show that behavioral therapies make patients too dependent on the staff in nursing homes. On the other hand, other studies show that behavioral therapies can improve a patient's ability to remember recent events when they are taken out of their routines.

Furthermore, behavioral therapies have also been used with patients who had noisemaking issues. In this respect, studies have shown that some dementia patients that used to have issues with noise making were able to overcome this symptom thanks to the behavioral interventions made by the therapists which reinforced quiet behavior in patients.

At the same time, it is important to note that patients dealing with dementia may sometimes make noise for reasons different than those related directly to the illness. They may be in pain, they may be trying to echo outside noise, or they may want to attract attention. An experienced therapist can distinguish between these situations and situations where noise making is part of the behavioral changes patients may experience.

Dementia Sensory Stimulation

Reduced sensory input can be a symptom experienced by patients with dementia. There are a few causes that may lead to this. In some instances, for example, the sensory acuity is deteriorated. In other instances, the patient's environment might be too monotonous and it may lack sensory stimulation. There are also instances when the person suffering from dementia might withdraw, which might also lead or be connected to external stimulation (this usually happens when patients have to cope with an unwanted experience, such as a noisy group of people surrounding them).

A lack of stimulation can lead to confusion, wandering, and other similar symptoms. Furthermore, it has also been shown that in some cases, patients with dementia may experience reduced anxiety levels when expressive physical touches, associated with verbalization, are used in the communication with them.

Many programs meant to help people suffering from dementia (and their loved ones) include social stimulation, psychosocial stimulation, and physical stimulation, because these have been shown to have positive effects on how the patient feels. Sometimes, these stimulation techniques include domestic activities or recreational activities, because these types of actions can stimulate the patients.

As with all the other therapies presented here, it is important that this, too, is employed by a professional who knows very well what they are doing. This needs to be well controlled to show results.

Motor Activity

A lot of programs that offer to help patients with dementia might also include motor activities. Unless the patient is too old or too frail, you should expect to see therapies in this general area in most of the aiding programs.

The reason motor activity therapies are so popular is because they have been linked to cognitive improvement. While the research is not conclusive when it comes to this, it is also important to note that motor activities can still be helpful.

Physical exercise can reduce weakening in the physical state of the patient. Also, some studies may suggest that physical exercise can improve not only the physical state of the patients, but also the cognitive state. Ideally, physical exercise should be performed during daytime, because doing this will improve the quality of their sleep as well.

Individual Psychotherapy

No doubt, individual psychotherapy is one of the most important (and widespread) therapies used in the management of a wide range of mental disorders. It may not be the case with dementia, though.

Although interest in working with the elderly has experienced a surge in popularity in more recent years, psychotherapy for patients with dementia is less frequent than in the case of mental disorder patients. For patients with dementia, this type of therapy is often used in combination with psychoeducational work with the families, and it comes to complement medication administration.

One of the reasons psychotherapy was not as commonly used in patients with dementia is the illness itself and how it may cause a lot of patients to be unaware of their own selves, making psychotherapy itself difficult.

Outside of the dementia spectrum, psychotherapy tends to be introspective and it relies a lot on the communication between the patient and the therapist. However, given the nature of this illness and the fact that many of the patients do not communicate beyond basic topics, and given that even if they *can* be introspective, this could trigger bad memories in their lives, introspective psychotherapy is not as widely used in the treatment and management of dementia.

Narrative psychotherapy with a focus on enhancing the cognitive abilities, narrative techniques, and group therapy have been shown to yield good results. The main purpose of this therapy in the case of patients with dementia is not so much to help them look within and discover certain parts of themselves, but to help them cope with depression and anxiety (both of which are commonly associated with dementia).

Therapeutic Buildings

The environment surrounding patients with dementia can have a big influence on how their illness evolves. The environment around people has been shown to affect the way they feel even when they are perfectly healthy - so, in the case of dementia patients, it can bear an even more important role.

The reason the environment is so important in these situations is because it helps the patient feel more secure in their ability to be as independent as possible. The better the environment is structured, the easier the patient will be able to build routines around it, to set up triggers to help them remember important things, and to feel generally less confused and disoriented.

In terms of how the building environment of a dementia patient should be created, it is revealing to say that it should be created the same way as it would be for an incapacitated person. In the case of people suffering from dementia, the main handicaps they have are characterized by impaired reasoning, impaired learning abilities, impaired memory, stress, and even a very sensitive way of perceiving the environment (both the social one and the built one).

Therefore, the design of the space in which a patient with dementia lives should focus on compensating for their disability. It should enable the patient to live as independently as possible, to feel self-confident, and to have a sense of self-esteem.

Some of the features of such a space include a relatively small size, a sense of familiarity and comfort, the presence of tools that help the patient live a normal life (to eat, to wash their clothes, to relax), different rooms for different functions, keeping the furniture in the place age-appropriate, adding different types of cues around the space (such as light, smell, or sounds), and so on.

The Improvement of the Quality of Life

Dementia can have a tremendous impact not only on the patient himself/herself, but also on the family and the community surrounding them.

One of the biggest impacts it has on the patient from their perspective is related to the fact that they may start to perceive their position in life differently.

At a general level, quality of life has three main levels: that of the subjective well-being, objective functioning, and the environmental living conditions. All of these levels are related to the cognitive status of the person affected (in this case, the patient suffering from Alzheimer's Disease or dementia). Since cognitive functions are precisely what are most affected in these cases, the support system around the patient (family, friends, therapists, therapy groups, and so on) should help the patient keep all the three levels of the quality of life at their highest.

As someone supporting a patient with dementia, knowing what to expect from the development of the illness in relation to the quality of life elements mentioned above will help you manage the situation better and help the ones you love. More specifically:

- In terms of subjective well-being, dementia patients can experience difficulty, frustration, denial, anxiety, depression, and negative emotions connected to the cognitive impairment they notice developing.
- In terms of objective functioning, some patients may experience trouble doing simple things (such as going out of the house and coming back, recognizing the ones they love, and so on).
- In terms of the environmental living conditions, everything should be adapted to the new "normal" in the patient's life. As mentioned in the previous section, the environment surrounding a patient with dementia should be altered in a way that helps them move past their impairment and handicaps. Otherwise, a sheltered environment with personal care services at the patient's disposal may be a better alternative.

There are multiple ways the quality of life can be improved for patients, and these can help them live fairly independently for longer. Changes and alterations will have to be made on multiple levels for the life of a patient suffering with dementia to be maintained at a good quality.

It is important that these changes are made only after a thorough discussion between the patient's caregiver and their doctor(s). Sometimes, small things that may seem normal to someone who is healthy might not function well for patients diagnosed with dementia. Therefore, the person caring for a dementia patient should document everything themselves and ask all the questions they need in order to make sure they are making the right decisions for their loved one.

What Will You and Your Loved Ones Lose - And Won't You?

Undoubtedly, a diagnosis of dementia brings with it a series of changes in one's life - and in the lives of the loved ones surrounding them. Your friends and family will have questions, as I am certain you had questions when learning about your diagnosis, too.

One of the most important underlying inquiries will be related to *how* exactly your life and their lives will change over the course of the next years - or, in other words, what you will lose and what you will not lose.

What You Will Lose

It would be unfair to you and your loved ones to say that nothing will change in a negative way - because it will, and it is important to be prepared from all points of view. Among the things that will slowly start to disappear from your life, the following are included:

Your Memory

Dementia and especially Alzheimer's Disease primarily affect the memory and the cognitive abilities. You will become more forgetful over time, and that is why it's important that those around you help you with this. If you decide not to be taken to a caregiving home, your home carer will have to help you by setting up memory triggers for you and helping you remember the important things.

Motor Skills

Motor skill problems are common across the entire dementia spectrum, but they are more common with some types of dementia. For instance, patients with frontotemporal dementia are less likely to experience memory issues in the early stages. However, in the later stages of the development of dementia, the symptoms will become more poignant - confusion, forgetfulness, swallowing issues, as well as motor skills will occur.

It is important to note that the loss of the fine motor skills is not a symptom of dementia only. In dementia, however, it appears to be more frequent in the case of Parkinson's disease patients, as well as Alzheimer's patients.

For instance, Alzheimer's disease patients might find it difficult to do things with their hands - including neat writing, tying shoelaces, or threading a needle.

The reason motor skills are connected to Alzheimer's (and dementia in general) is because some tasks are automatically stored within our so called "muscle memory." Things you have learned early on, like tying your shoelaces for example, and which have become automatic are usually included on that "side" of the memory.

Sometimes, motor skills are lost when the connection between the brain and the muscles is damaged. Some studies have even shown that changes in gait (e.g. taking shorter steps when walking) can be an early sign of the disease.

In the case of Parkinson's Disease and Alzheimer's disease, another cause for motor skill problems can be the numbness patients experience in their extremities.

The Remembering Self

According to Daniel Kahneman[10], people view experiences in two main ways: through the prism of something called the "experiential self" (which deals with all the things related to living) or through the prism of something called the "remembering self" (which deals with storing what the experiential self has recorded).

Kahneman gives a very good explanation on this by correlating the understanding of the experiential self and the remembering self with two couples going on vacation. The first, the experiential self representatives, will just go on vacation for the experience itself, and they might not even bring along a camera. The second, however, will want to remember everything and they will take a lot of pictures, no matter what.

In the case of Alzheimer's disease patients, as well as patients suffering from other types of dementia, the experiential self will not go away. However, the remembering self will start to disappear, along with the memory.

Remembering the distinction between the remembering self and the experiential self becomes crucial in the way caregivers tend to dementia patients. Sometimes, they might not emphasize the quality of care as much, doing brusque things and maybe even being un-courteous towards the person suffering from dementia, precisely because they think the patient will not remember it anyway.

However, it is extremely important to keep in mind the fact that although that person might not "record" the memory by taking a mental "photograph" of it, they will still experience the bad moment. Therefore, it will still make them feel bad, even though they might not remember it later on.

Learning to live with a patient with dementia in a way that allows them to experience the best of the present is very important. It is, in the end, quite crucial to making sure the patient will still maintain a sense of self, even if just for the absolute "present."

Rational Thinking

Unfortunately, dementia affects rational thinking to the point where the most advanced patients cannot be reasoned with in any way.

Impaired decision-making is relatively common throughout the entire spectrum of dementia. Sooner or later, this symptom affects all those diagnosed with dementia, regardless of whether it's Alzheimer's, Lewy Bodies, or Frontotemporal dementia.

As was mentioned earlier in the book, a patient diagnosed with dementia should consider the fact that, at some point in the development of the illness, they might not be able to make legal decisions - so they should prepare all the paperwork before that

---

[10]Memory Vs. Experience: Happiness is Relative. (2019). Retrieved from https://www.psychologicalscience.org/observer/memory-vs-experience-happiness-is-relative

moment occurs.

Most of the studies on how the decision making process degradates in patients with dementia has focused on reasoning deficits and some executive functions. However, more recent research has pointed out that there are a variety of neuropsychological processes that contribute to decision-making in general (including processes that are connected to reward and punishment). However, it is very important to note that these components are not necessarily recognized in legal environments (and sometimes, they are not recognized in medical environments either).

What You Will Not Lose

Fortunately, dementia does not take *everything* away from you and your family. Some sides of your life will not change (or not as much), and it is important to focus on these, as they will give you a sense of balance and dignity (both as a patient and as a caregiver).

Unfortunately, the things a dementia patient will not lose are not always on the positive side - and this makes it utterly important for the caretaker to understand them and to know how to react to them, because improving these parts of a dementia patient's life can help them improve the overall quality of their life.

Feelings

Although patients diagnosed with dementia might have less control over how they express their feelings, they most definitely *do* experience changes in how they respond emotionally.

Unfortunately, it is not always the best emotions that surface in the case of dementia patients. Sometimes, their negative feelings become uncontrollable and they become irritable, they might change their mood very rapidly, or they might be uninterested and distant towards different things brought forward to them.

These are some of the most difficult parts to deal with as a caregiver. However, as a caretaker, you should always remind yourself that these behaviors are caused by brain damage. Very often, patients with dementia may become very emotional in situations that scare them - such as remembering disappearing memories or feeling unable to think clearly in situations they know they have dealt with before. Sometimes, these strong emotions are caused by needs that are not fulfilled - and this is something the caretaker can actually help with, because once they've identified those needs, fulfilling them should bring a little more balance for the patient.

Confidence

Sometimes, people suffering from dementia might feel insecure, or they might lose their confidence and self-esteem because they realize that their abilities have been diminished. When they feel that they cannot be in control anymore, they might find it difficult to trust their own judgment. On top of this, some patients with dementia might feel the effects of the social stigma that comes with this poorly understood diagnosis.

Sometimes, patients with dementia might feel a loss in self-esteem as an indirect cause. For instance, if someone's financial status, employment status, or relationships will be affected by the diagnosis, they might suffer and lose confidence and self-esteem.

On the other hand, there are also people who form new relationships after finding out their diagnosis, because they come in contact with people suffering from the same illness as part of different classes or support groups. In these cases, these groups can actually help one regain their self-confidence by helping them feel less alone in this journey.

As a partner and/or main caretaker, it is extremely important for you to help the dementia patient maintain their self-esteem at higher levels. Some of the things you could do include the following:

- Always praise and encourage them, regardless of how small their successes may be
- Always focus on the positive
- Don't criticize too hard
- Don't make belittling comments
- Help them do the activities they enjoy (and which help give them purpose)
- Help them maintain social relationships
- Help them form new social relationships

Dementia patients will not automatically lose their self-confidence as a direct result of the illness. They will slowly grow into this as the aforementioned problems might appear in their lives. As a caretaker, it is of the utmost importance that you support your loved one in this situation and that you stand by their side.

Enjoying Beauty and Life

Although life as a dementia patient is not easy by any standard, this doesn't mean that people suffering from Alzheimer's or other forms of dementia will not find beauty in living.

On the contrary, people suffering from dementia might find enjoyment sooner than a healthy person. For instance, if your entire family decides to go on vacation, the patient with dementia will most likely be the happiest. Furthermore, persons with dementia might find even more happiness in the things they love than they used to when they were healthy (e.g. some patients will be genuinely happy listening to the same beloved song over and over again).

Yes, dementia can come as a strike of lighting for everyone involved: patients, family, friends, and caretakers. However, focusing on the positives is very important because it will help you and your loved to live a more fulfilling life in general.

Sensory Feedback

Although sensory feedback is related to the brain, it is one of the things a patient diagnosed with dementia will not actually lose. Every part of their body is connected to the brain the same way it is with everyone else. The nerves in the human body (e.g. the gustatory nerves) do not process information on their own - they just momentarily store it before sending it to the brain, where it can handle them and "reinterpret" them.

Whenever the senses are stimulated, the brain is stimulated - and this is good for patients with dementia because it helps them stay in tune with their bodies and it plain and simply makes them happier.

A beautiful landscape, a good meal, a nice perfume, a song they love, or simply a gentle touch from someone familiar - these things can make a difference in how patients with dementia experience their illness. This can make them a little happier and a little more able to cope with what is going on with them.

There are five senses that are usually known, as well as two less recognized senses that are sometimes associated with dementia patients:

- Sight - experienced through the eyes, the sense through which most people gain most of their information
- Hearing - experienced through the ears, providing humans with a very vibrant source of stimulation
- Smell - experienced through the nose, one of the senses most associated with memories
- Taste - experienced through the nerve endings on the tongue, one of the most pleasurable senses
- Touch - experienced through the receptors on the human skin, one of the easier senses to stimulate because anything that touches us will be stimulating

- Proprioceptive stimulation - a sense that is frequently hard to define and is related to informing the brain where some parts of the body are. For instance, a stroll through the park will stimulate the visual sense (through the nice view), the olfactory sense (through the smells), the auditory sense (through the natural sounds combined with those made by humans), and the proprioceptive sense (through the exercise of walking, which reminds the brain where different parts of the body are)
- Vestibular stimulation - a sense connected to the proprioceptive system that allows our brain to establish physical balance, as well as stand and move without falling. This sense is connected to the auditory, tactile, and visual systems.

Fight or Flight

A lot of the people diagnosed with dementia become angry (sometimes out of the blue without no apparent reason). Agitation, upset, and fright are common emotions experienced by those with dementia.

Many times, this type of anger might appear to be directed the caretaker as a result of them doing something wrong. However, this is related to the so-called "fight or flight" response dementia patients experience.

To understand why this response appears, think again about the fact that in the case of someone diagnosed with dementia, they cannot perceive the reality around them correctly - and this sometimes includes situations that might feel threatening to the patient.

Many times, this response is triggered by actions that are nothing less than innocent. However, the reaction of the dementia sufferer might feel over the top because their brains are simply not wired to perceive threats correctly anymore.

To be more specific: there are two sources from which the brain can "draw" information into the amygdala - through the thalamus (the direct route) or through the thalamus and the cortex (the indirect route).

When the information is delivered using the first channel (through the thalamus), the brain might release a fight or flight response.

On the other hand, when the information travels through the indirect channel, it allows for more evaluation, helping the brain determine if a situation is threatening or not.

In the case of people suffering from dementia, the parts of the brain that normally deal with the perception of threats are deteriorated. As a result of this, very normal and innocent actions (such as a caretaker wanting to feed the patient) will be perceived as threatening situations by the dementia patient.

There are some things you can do to avoid this kind of fight or flight response:

- Always be friendly when approaching the person
- Smile when both approaching the person and when communicating with them
- If necessary, remind the person who you are by presenting your name and telling them about your relationship
- Be respectful
- Reassure the person
- Use a low voice (it is less likely to be perceived as threat this way)
- Try to limit potential interferences, such as the TV or the radio
- Don't use complicated sentences and words; be as simple as possible
- Speak to the person by making same level eye contact, even if they are sitting
- Assume a gentle, affectionate attitude
- Before you start talking, make sure you have the patient's attention.

If the patient becomes angry or agitated as a result of a fight or flight response, it is essential that you react correctly:

- Change the subject as soon as possible
- Change the environment (e.g. take the patient for a walk), but do make sure you inform the person about this first in a kind tone, without rushing them
- Touch them in a non invasive, gentle way
- Change the tone of your voice and speak soothingly
- Remind the patient of a happy memory
- Ensure that the patient is not surrounded by any kind of dangerous object
- Do *not* restrain them physically
- Show sympathy and empathy

Knowing what to expect as a patient with dementia, as well as a caretaker, is very important. Things are not going to be easy, but being prepared will help you stay stronger for the ones you love, regardless of which "side" you are on: the patient or the caretaker.

In the following section, I will present you with situations that are quite common in real life and how you can use our examples to help your loved one live a generally better life.

Common Situations and How to Deal with Them

Helping a patient who suffers from dementia might prove to be very difficult, depending on how advanced the disease is. The reason helping the patient with dementia is so difficult is because the illness makes them unable to reason. Therefore, if they don't want to do something, they might just not do it.

Some of the most common real-life situations will be included in this section, with a very important note: the manners by which we are suggesting these things to be treated are just that, suggestions. Read about them, analyze them, and talk to your doctor if something seems too off, or you have noticed something that is wrong.

Making The Patient Feel Useful

There are three signs that show a person suffering from dementia feels like they have a purpose:

- They make genuine efforts to be part of the activities they are involved in
- They accept daily chores and activities happily
- They are trying hard to complete tasks and activities as well as they can

On the other hand, some of the main obstacles that might stand between a dementia patient and purposefulness are helplessness, lacking identity, lacking self-worth, and boredom - all of which take on a chronic-like state in the lives of those suffering with dementia.

There are some activities that can help you make a person with dementia happy, but the most popular ones include the following:

- Crafts - it doesn't have to be something complicated; a simple project will do. For instance, you can engage the patient in making a cushion table or creating a beaded bracelet.
- Chores - this will help the person suffering from dementia feel like less of a

burden and it will help them feel useful again. It will also help them feel that they have a sense of purpose.

- Sorting - this is a relatively easy task, but it will help the dementia patient feel like they can help and have a purpose. For instance, you could give them a drawer full of photos or even socks and ask the patient to sort the objects there according to different rules (e.g. by color, by theme, etc.)

Although they might not seem like much, these activities can make a world of difference for the dementia patient, especially since lack of purpose and depression can be two of the most common and most awful symptoms of dementia.

Enabling Communication

Communication lies at the very basis of a healthy human being - and at the very basis of a healthy relationship as well. Encouraging a patient to talk, especially to other people who are going through the same thing, can make a very big difference.

Do keep in mind that enabling communication for a person with dementia involves both verbal communication and non-verbal communication (such as the gestures, body language, and so on).

When communicating with a person who suffers from dementia, your verbal communication and your non-verbal gestures should coordinate. In other words, what you say should coordinate with your gestures, your tone, your face, and so on. This will help the person at the receiving end of the message understand you even if their cognitive abilities are flawed by their illness.

When you are having a discussion with a dementia patient, it is very important to prepare the environment and to set the right ambiance for this. Namely, you should:

1. Reduce any kind of background noise. For persons suffering from dementia, focusing is an issue regardless of the environment. If there is some sort of background noise happening, the confusion may be even higher. For instance, car traffic, TV sounds, or even a vacuum cleaner in a different room can interrupt the communication process and lower your chances of actually sending your message across. Therefore, you should make sure to remove any kind of source of noise and distractions that might affect the person you are communicating with.

2. Take it slow. Since the person suffering from dementia might go at a much slower pace than you do in everyday communication, it is important to adjust to that. Relax your body and your mind and remove any kind of tension at every level before you start discussing with the patient.

3. Consider the emotional state. It is quite important to know how the person

suffering from dementia is feeling at the moment. If they are anxious or distressed, frightened, angry, or frustrated, they might not react well to opening the communication channel.

4. Consider the illness. One of the primary symptoms of dementia is memory loss. In some cases, the short term memory loss might get so bad that, as a caretaker, every encounter with the person suffering from dementia might feel like the first time, even if you have already met them several times that day.
5. Greet the person. It is important to introduce yourself correctly when opening the discussion channel with a person suffering from dementia. Otherwise, they might not recognize you and a "fight or flight" response may be triggered. Be warm and friendly when giving your greetings to create a comfortable atmosphere between the two of you.
6. Take the right physical approach. Sometimes, people suffering from dementia are withdrawn and they may be startled when someone enters their physical space. Do this gently by keeping your eyes at their level. If the person is very distracted, you might want to spend some time alongside them, making minimal movements, so that they can get accustomed to you being there.
7. Analyze the emotional state. Is the person happy? This could be a good conversation starter. Also, the emotion the patient has when responding to physical touch (e.g. a reassuring hand on the back) can also tell you more about the state they are in. If they reject the touch, you should tread carefully when doing this the next time. If, on the other hand, they clasp your hand, it might be a sign they need more support.
8. Constantly check in and analyze the emotional responses of the interlocutor. This is valid in any kind of communication, but it grows in importance with dementia patients. You want to make sure that they feel good throughout the communication process and that no discomfort is caused to them. The tone of their voice and how it changes, the facial expressions, the body position - they can tell a lot about whether or not you should proceed with the conversation onwards.
9. Know that sometimes, a simple conversation may trigger a flood of emotions. People suffering from dementia frequently experience very powerful emotions. Sometimes, they are positive - like laughter. Other times, they might be triggered to remember painful memories and experience anxiety and grief. Be there regardless of what emotions might come to surface and offer them your support - they need this more than anything else.
10. If you notice an emotional reaction, say it out loud. This will help the other

person see that you care about them. For instance, if you have noticed that the patient has withdrawn or that they look sad, you could tell them "You look saddened." Do the same with positive emotions, too!

11. Be flexible. No matter how many scenarios you make up in your mind before striking up a conversation with the patient, things might still take a different turn. Be ready for that. Also, be ready to deal with a limited content of speech, and not just from a linguistic point of view. For instance, for a person with dementia, all women may be a Mary - so, in conversation, they might refer to all the women they know and remember as "Mary."

12. Understand their reality. If you are a loved one, you are more than familiar with the past and present of the person suffering from dementia. Use your key information to interpret the meaning behind some of the more cryptic sentences said by the person on the other end of the communication string.

13. Cling on to every detail to keep the talk going. When communicating with a person who suffers from dementia, listening is more important than ever. Knowing how to spot a connection will help you keep the conversation going, and it will help the other person stimulate their brain as well. Things like using the other person's name, acknowledging that you understood what they are saying, and so on can make the communication smoother.

14. Don't confront them. It is not only pointless, but it will create agitation and anger in the interlocutor as well. Also, if they make mistakes (such as not telling the time correctly), analyze their emotional state before you do anything. Also, don't simply tell them that they made a mistake - suggest to them the right answer in a non-confrontational way (e.g. "It looks like it's 10 am outside, the sun is up and everyone is having their breakfasts, what do you think?").

15. Don't keep the conversation going for too long. It might become fatiguing for the other person, and when that happens, anxiety and agitation might crop up as well. Keep the discussions short, but frequent.

16. Finish the conversation correctly as well. If you are leaving the room, be sure the person knows it. If you are leaving their house, be sure they know it and that you bid your farewell. If you think you will return at some point during the day to check up on them, do make sure you tell them that.

Moreover, make sure you have the other person's attention. Be friendly and smile just like when you started the conversation, and be polite by letting them know that you have enjoyed the time spent with them.

17. Consider the Talking Mats. Sometimes, people suffering from dementia have very

limited verbal skills. In these cases, you might need Talking Mats - interactive systems consisting of cards with pictures that help people with disabilities learn easier. Sometimes, they are used by patients with dementia so that they have something to point to.

Running Errands with People with Dementia

If a person has dementia in a more advanced state, running errands with them can be difficult because they are prone to getting angry, confused, or irritated due to all the sounds and the unstructured surroundings they are experiencing.

Therefore, if you have to run errands with someone who suffers from dementia, you should make sure the person is getting both sensory and social stimulation. In other words, you should try to search the beautiful parts and show them to the other person, and you should also make sure to focus as much as you can on the person, rather than the task.

This might sound ambiguous, but once you learn the basics of communicating and behaving around a person with dementia, you will understand. For instance, focusing on the person is all about making this errand all about them - telling them that you are going to have fun, speaking about the emotional triggers you may notice, and so on.

Furthermore, searching for the beautiful parts is all about stimulating the other person to see the nice things. It might be a cloudless sky, the colors of the leaves, or simply the fact that you are both together, enjoying yourselves.

Dealing with Delusions

Although not *everyone* who suffers from dementia will experience delusions, many will, particularly in the case of Alzheimer's Disease. Of all the symptoms usually associated with dementia, delusions are the most confusing and downright terrifying, both for the patient and for the caretaker as well.

To someone who has not dealt with this type of symptom in particular, they might seem like pure and simple movie scenarios. But for dementia patients and their loved ones, delusions become a new "normal" - one where the face of a beloved wife is juxtaposed on the face of the mother, aunt, or neighbor, and no delineation is made between the two persons.

There are a few medical conditions that connect dementia and delusions:

1. Capgras Syndrome: First described in 1923 by a psychiatrist with the same name, Capgras Syndrome makes the patient believe that someone familiar in their lives has been replaced by a "duplicate," a person who might look the same, but has evil intentions. This condition is not correlated with dementia only, as it can be

seen in schizophrenia, epilepsy, cerebrovascular disease, and traumatic injuries.

2. Fregoli Syndrome: This condition is named after an actor who was famous in the 1920s for his impersonation skills. Patients who suffer from this syndrome frequently mistake unfamiliar places and people and familiar ones.

3. Reduplicative Paramnesia: This was described at the beginning of the 20th century by Arnold Pick. People suffering from this condition think that some of the people they meet are “clones” who look the same, but are different in terms of personality and behavior.

These delusions are common in people who suffer from dementia, and one of the explanations people have given for them is that the right hemisphere of the brain, in charge of “familiarity” can be affected in some dementia patients. Sometimes, the frontal lobe lesions might be implicated in the process as well.

Even more specifically, it appears that the perirhinal cortex, a region of the brain, is underactive in the case of Capgras syndrome (case in which the patient is uncertain of the familiarity), but overactive in the case of the Fregoli syndrome (case in which the patient has a false sense of familiarity).

People affected by these syndromes will find it very difficult to explain the sense of confusion or how it is that their sense of familiarity is completely out of context.

Beyond the confusion and unsettling emotions these syndromes generate, the complications of suffering from them can be severe. A wife can flee the house in the middle of the night, convinced that her true husband has been replaced by a fake one. Some people might go as far as homicide in the case of the Capgras syndrome.

People suffering from the Fregoli syndrome can become dangerous to others and to themselves as well, when they might mistake a complete stranger for a familiar person they don’t like or fear.

And in the case of those suffering from reduplicative paramnesia, the stress of trying to determine which of the “two” familiar people is the real one and who is the imposter can be unnerving at the very least.

Given how dangerous and stressful these conditions can be, immediate treatment must be sought to ensure the safety of both the patient and those around them.

There are some forms of treatment that help in these cases:

1. Habilitation therapy. This type of therapy comes in addition to other therapies people with dementia might be undergoing. It is extremely important that these are used because, like in most of the psychotic conditions, the first type of

treatment that is tried should be the non-medicated one.

The reason behind this is connected to the fact that trying to tell a delusional person that their fears are unfounded and untrue can be extremely difficult. Instead of doing this and forcing the truth down on patients suffering from delusional conditions, habilitation therapy enters the world of the patient and acknowledges their fears to re-mold the entire delusional field into a positive experience, rather than a frightening one.

In this type of therapy, nobody tries to convince the patient that they are wrong. For instance, if an "imposter" is present in the room, they will go out and return with a friendly smile and warm voice that will trigger positive feelings in the person suffering from delusions.

2. Medication. When the safety of the patient and those around them is in danger, medication may be tried. The medication treatment available for such conditions is based on cognitive enhancers, antidepressants, and antipsychotics. Unfortunately, though, none of the options can *treat* the condition. In the case of cognitive enhancers, the amelioration of the behavioral symptoms is considered to be limited. In the case of some antidepressants prescribed in these situation, the success reported is only anecdotal. And in the case of antipsychotic medication, success has been reported only in some cases (plus, it must be noted that these drugs come with a death risk warning for those who suffer from dementia and psychosis).

Delusions *can* be treated by using the right attitude, compassion, patience, the correct therapies, and, sometimes, some medication. However, drugs are usually the last option for the list of reasons mentioned above - so the most important elements of dealing with delusions in dementia patients remain your attitude as a caretaker and the care given.

Traveling with a Dementia Patient

A dementia diagnosis does not necessarily mean the patient cannot travel (accompanied by their caretaker, of course). However, before making the decision to take them on a trip, it is important to assess their symptoms and see if they are able to do this.

This is extremely important because some patients might be doing quite well in their familiar environment, but once out, their symptoms might worsen. Particularly, symptoms like wandering, anger outbursts, or agitation could reach higher levels when the patient is taken out of their familiar comfort zone. This is connected to the fact that, in the case of people suffering from dementia, routine and familiarity create a sense of security - all of which turns to nothing when the patient is taken out of the space he/she is familiar with.

The signs that traveling with dementia might not be a safe choice include the following:

- The patient suffers from dementia in the later stage
- The patient is frequently confused, agitated, and disoriented even in the most familiar spaces
- The patient is upset by loud environments
- The patient is at risk of falling and hurting themselves
- The patient cannot manage their incontinence properly
- The patient constantly wants to return home when they are out of the house or visiting someone
- The patient wanders
- The patient experiences delusions, paranoia, or inappropriate behavior
- The patient yells, screams, or cries without any apparent reason
- The patient is physically or verbally aggressive
- The patient suffers from medical conditions that are unstable

If your loved one does not fall in the aforementioned categories, they might be able to travel with you. If the person suffering from dementia does not meet the aforementioned criteria, ask yourself the following questions to determine if, even outside of these behaviors and situations, the patient can still undergo the stress and the unfamiliarity of traveling.

1. How advanced are their dementia symptoms?

Most of the time, patients diagnosed with early stage dementia can still travel. However, as the illness progresses, they might find it difficult and overwhelming.

If your loved one suffers from middle stage dementia, the decision on whether or not you should take them away with you when traveling can be difficult. It is extremely important to be very realistic when assessing their challenges, especially since symptoms can be fleeting and varied. Generally, when it comes to this matter, it is better to be safe than sorry.

Unfortunately, patients with later stage dementia are not recommended to travel. At this point, the illness has already fatigued the patient and they are most likely overwhelmed by simple, everyday activities, they are more vulnerable to catching other types of diseases and infections, and they might have problems eating, swallowing, or even sitting.

2. How are you dealing with your loved one's situation?

There are two ends of the dementia diagnosis: the person suffering from it and the person(s) around the patient. Even if the patient is dealing well with their symptoms and they might not be in a very advanced stage of the disease, it is still very important to assess whether *you* are ready to travel with them or not.

This is extremely important, because traveling with someone who suffers from dementia is not easy in any way, not even for someone who already has experience in caring for a person with this diagnosis. Even with all the planning in the world, you might still have to deal with unexpected situations, such as challenging behaviors (which might sometimes happen in public), sleep deprivation, and situations that are extremely stressful.

If you are dealing well with the current symptoms of dementia shown by your loved one, and if they are not very advanced in their illness, you can travel with them. However, if you are struggling to deal with their symptoms at the moment, if you are feeling very tired and overwhelmed, or if you are generally new at dealing with the symptoms, traveling with a patient suffering from dementia might not be the best idea.

3. Are they OK with crowded and loud environments?

You may not fully know how someone with dementia will react when they are facing a crowded space that is unfamiliar. However, how they react when they are out in public might be a good indicator of this. If you know that their behavior can become uncontrollable in certain public environments, such as restaurants, malls, or grocery stores, it is likely that traveling with them might not be a good idea.

Even if they don't react extremely to these kinds of spaces, if you know that it makes them feel uncomfortable, tired, angry, anxious, or terrified, putting them in the situation of dealing with a public space that is completely unknown to them is not a good idea - and thus, traveling with them might not be exactly OK either.

4. Do you really have to take this trip?

While traveling can be fun, it is worth considering the risks of going away with someone who suffers from dementia. Even if their behavior back home is good, there is still a margin of unpredictability you should definitely take into consideration.

Given the situation, think thoroughly: is it worth taking this trip? For instance, if you are traveling to attend a family event that is meaningful for the patient with dementia, it might be worth taking the risk (provided that the patient meets all the criteria, as mentioned above). However, a trip that is made just for fun might not be as worth it.

5. What is the destination?

Places that are already familiar for someone who suffers from dementia might be easier to travel to. For instance, if you travel to a place your loved one used to go to often before they developed the illness, they might find it easier to adapt to that location.

Furthermore, you should try to only travel to places that allow you to keep the patient's routine as intact as possible.

Last, but not least, the *means* by which you travel can have a huge influence as well. For example, traveling by car will most likely give you more flexibility. However, traveling by plane tends to be a bit more chaotic, and thus, more likely to generate unexpected situations. If you have to travel by air, try to keep the flight as short as possible and to avoid airport transfers, as these can be unnerving for a person with dementia (it can be stressful for anyone, not to mention someone who doesn't fully understand what is going on).

6. Will you be the only one tending to the patient with dementia?

Handling an adult who suffers from dementia all on your own when you are away from home can be very difficult, especially given the fact that it can be a very unpredictable situation overall. If you are taking another caretaker with you, the situations that might arise will be easier to handle.

If you have decided that traveling with your loved one suffering from dementia should be OK, do ensure that you follow these tips to make sure the trip is safe:

- Opt for familiar destinations. As mentioned before, these locations are usually easier to handle for someone who is confused and whose memory is affected by dementia.

- Be prepared for the fact that, even with all the planning in the world, traveling may still be confusing and chaotic for a person suffering from dementia.

- Be prepared for the fact that any change in the environment might trigger the ill person to wander. This might be true for people in the early stages of dementia as well. It is better to take precautions, like enrolling the dementia patient in different tracking systems that will allow you to find them if they wander.

- If you will be traveling long-term, you should consider contacting the Alzheimer's Association at local level. They might be able to provide you with resources and support, particularly if you are traveling within the borders of the United States.

- Always carry a bag with you to include the medications, the travel itinerary, some change of clothes, snacks, activities for the dementia patient, and water.

- Do make sure you pack the patient's medication, their most up to date medical information, copies of the legal documents, as well as a list of the most important emergency contacts.
- Take your time to create an itinerary with minute details of each destination. Share this itinerary with your emergency contacts back home as well and carry a copy of the itinerary with you all the time.
- Inform the hotel staff that you might have specific needs
- Avoid traveling at night, as this might cause confusion for a person suffering with dementia whose normal routine is to sleep at night
- Some of the most important documents you should absolutely make sure to pack away include the following: the names of the doctors assisting your loved one and their contact information, a list of the medications the patient is taking at the moment and their dosages, all the phone numbers of the local police, fire departments, hospitals, and emergency institutions (including poison control)
- A list of allergies
- Copies of any important legal papers - such as the living will, the advanced directives, the power of attorney, and so on
- The names of your emergency contacts back home
- Insurance number and name

If you decide to travel by air (or if you simply have no other choice), it is important to prepare yourself for doing this alongside someone who suffers from dementia. The crowds in airports, the constant buzz, and the general level of social interaction can all have a negative impact on someone diagnosed with dementia.

Also, if you have to travel by air, here are some tips for you to keep in mind:

- You should avoid stressful flights that have very tight connections, as these might put too much stress on the patient suffering from dementia.
- Do consider asking for a wheelchair, even if the patient can use his/her motor skills correctly. This will give you the assurance that you will be able to move through the airport without having to face unpleasant situations.
- Contact TSA (the Transportation Security Administration) within about 3 days

before traveling to ask for information on what to expect for the security screening. Also, when this is happening, try to remind the person suffering from dementia about what this process involves. Consider telling the security agent about the diagnosis of the person you are accompanying as well.

- Don't be afraid to ask for help from in-flight crew and airport employees.
- Stay with the dementia patient every second and don't let them out of sight. If possible, when they need to go to the restroom, choose the companion ones that will allow you to monitor them at all times.

Traveling with someone who has dementia is not easy, but it can be done as long as some basic criteria are met. However, as mentioned above as well, if the risks outweigh the benefits, think twice before booking your loved one a ticket, because the entire experience might turn out to be too frightening and stressful - both for the dementia patient and for you as well.

Dinner with Dementia Patients

Because dementia affects persons at such a grand scale, simple activities can become difficult for the person suffering from this illness, as well as the person(s) surrounding them.

Having dinner (and eating in general) should be incorporated in a very well-established routine if you want the patient to feel alright, if you want them to be able to eat and enjoy the food, and if you want to avoid unpleasant situations.

As a caretaker, there are several factors you should consider when it comes to eating with a dementia patient:

1. The dining environment. This can have a crucial importance on how well a patient with dementia eats. In general, aim for a relaxed, social surrounding that makes the patient feel comfortable and adds a sense of familiarity and structure to the day. Some of the following strategies might help:
    - Dedicate a special room for dining. This will help the patient develop a sense of familiarity, and once the routine has been established, they will always associate going to the dining room with meal time.
    - Try to set the dining room close to the kitchen. This will allow the aromas of the food to pass through and it might trigger a signal in the affected person's mind.
    - If you notice that your dear one is more comfortable eating in a different room, don't be afraid to make that the dining room. Every patient with

dementia is different and they may get triggered different ways.

- Do consider the fact that one meal can take up to one hour for a person suffering from dementia, so make them comfortable during this time.

2. Take your time preparing for meal time. Nothing in the life of a person suffering with dementia should be sudden - and this includes meal time as well. Some of the tips you might consider applying to make sure dinners are a success include the following:

    - Prepare the person for the dinner (or meal) ahead of them and take your time with this.
    - Take a short walk outside before the dinner, to encourage the patient's appetite.
    - If the person can handle it, encourage them to help you prepare for meal time. Things such as preparing the table for dinner can help trigger a signal that it is time to eat.
    - The sounds and smells of cooking can help the person remember that it is meal time.
    - Seat the person suffering from dementia in a way that makes them feel comfortable. For instance, if they like seeing other people when eating, make sure this always happens. Furthermore, if they might be distracted by what they see outside the window, try to position them with their face turned towards elements that will not distract them.
    - The actual physical comfort of the person matters a lot - so make sure the chair is comfortable and that the patient does not need to go to the bathroom before dinner time.
    - Make sure your loved one is fully ready to eat every time, with all the help they might need (e.g. make sure their glasses are on, that their dentures are clean and fit well, as well as make sure that their hearing aids are on if they need them).
    - Ensure the environment is very clean and soothing
    - Remove all distractions (including the TV, which should be turned off during the meal if it makes the person feel distracted).
    - Be sure the lighting allows the person to see everything on the table, including the food and the cutlery.

- It might be a good idea to remove the mirrors in the dining room, as this can create disorientation for someone suffering from dementia.
- Turn off any kind of noisy appliance in the house, including a washing machine that might be running in the background. Otherwise, this may be a source of noise and distraction.
- If the person suffering from dementia likes music, you can play it in the background.
- Do not rush through dinner. The general atmosphere should be relaxed and comforting. If difficulties arise, try to not add to the stress, as the dementia patient might sense this and they might become even more agitated and anxious.
- All the food on the plate should be visible, as the person might forget to eat it otherwise.
- Try not to remove the plates until everyone is done with their food. Otherwise, this might trigger a signal that meal time is over and the person diagnosed with dementia might not eat as much.
- Try not to get interrupted (even if it's by other people entering the room).
- Don't talk to other people, as the dementia patient might notice this and they might feel distracted by it.

3. Create the right setting. You need to make sure the person with dementia sees the table setting the same every time, and they have their own space to take their dinner. For instance, using a placement or a special tray will help them remember their place at the table. Furthermore, the following tactics will help as well:

   - The table setting should be as simple as possible. The fewer items on the table, the better it will be for the patient. Try to minimize this as much as possible by removing all objects that are not used during the actual dinner - and this might include the salt and pepper shakers, the condiments, the napkin holders, and so on.
   - You can keep a vase of flowers on the table because it can create a soothing, beautiful environment for some patients. However, if you notice that this is a distraction, remove it from the table at dinner time every time.
   - Try to use plates and bowls without patterns, because the dementia patient's perspective might be altered and they might find it difficult to tell the

difference between the two types of objects. Instead, try to use contrasting colors for the plates and the bowls, as this will help the patient distinguish between the two during meal time.

- Stick to primary colors, as they are easier to recognize. On the other hand, pastel colors might be difficult to process for patients with dementia because they might not see the difference between them.
- Use colored glasses because, again, they are easier to recognize.
- Keep the table linens simple. The patterned ones might cause the dementia patient to be distracted, as they will try to "pick" things off the tablecloth.
- Only lay utensils that are needed: the knife, the fork, and the spoon. Do not make it unnecessarily complicated for your loved one to tell the difference between the different types of utensils. Also, if the person prefers using a specific type of utensil (even though it is not the "traditional" one), use that instead of anything else. It's always best to make the person feel comfortable.

4. Eat with the person. Some people suffering from dementia might eat better if they are accompanied by someone else. The reason this happens is because it allows them to see a "model" they can copy. Also, the following tips will make dinner time more enjoyable and less eventful as well:

- Talk about the colors, flavors, and textures of the food, as this helps the patient be more stimulated (and thus, it helps the brain stay more active). It also helps the patient feel more comfortable with what is on their plate if they know exactly what each of the ingredients is and how it tastes.
- Encourage the person to eat independently whenever they can, but make sure you never make a comment on *how* they eat, as this might sadden or upset them.
- If you notice the person looks like they forgot what to do at meal time, prompt them by putting the cutlery in their hand.
- If the person is initiating eye contact, make sure you maintain it, as this means that they are seeking the comfort you can offer.
- Be prepared to aid with eating. As the illness progresses, the person suffering with dementia might need all of your help - including at meal time. If and when this happens, always treat them with dignity.
- If the hands are shaky or if the person loses control over the utensils, do use

an apron to protect their clothes.

- Always ask the person if the food is too hot or too cold

5. Consider their favorite time to eat. The key to keeping a dementia patient as happy as possible is molding their routine to the things they actually like doing, as this will provide them with a sense of independence and it might help them feel better. Therefore, you should prepare the main meal around the time the dementia patient is the hungriest, as this will help them feel better during the meal and it might help them eat better and more.

Furthermore, keep in mind the following food-related tips:

- Serve one course at a time, as serving multiple foods at once might create confusion for someone suffering from dementia
- Serving half-portions instead of full portions might help as well. However, try to keep the other half of the portion warm until the first one is gone.
- Try to avoid giving drinks to dementia persons during the actual meal. This can be confusing and distracting. Even more, drinks can be too filling and they might take the person off their meal.
- Use a wall clock that points out the time for breakfast, lunch, and dinner. This will help the person suffering from dementia know when it is time for a meal.

6. Make it a good meal every time. As it was mentioned earlier in this book, the sense of beauty and pleasure is not lost in dementia patients. Therefore, you should try and make every meal feel like a sensory stimulation, both visually and from the point of view of the smell and that of the taste.

Moreover, make sure you do these things as well:

- Remember that the food temperature should be just right. Sometimes, people suffering with dementia might not be able to tell if something is too hot.
- Always try to serve foods the patient liked before the onset of the disease. However, if they don't like those foods anymore, don't try to serve them insistently. Also, don't worry if your loved one might want to eat the same type of meal twice or even three times in a row - if it pleases them, it is more than OK.
- Try to make the plate as colorful as possible, as this will be more attractive and it will help the dementia patient distinguish between the different types of food on their plate. Furthermore, try to contrast between the color of the plates and the color of the food (for instance, it might be difficult for someone suffering from

dementia to distinguish between a poached egg and a white plate).

- Don't overload each plate with food, as this might feel overwhelming for the patient.
- Use cutlery that allows the person to be independent even if their coordination is poor.
- Because the meals might take longer than the usual, try to use insulated plates to keep the food warmer for longer.
- Use taller plates to keep the food from slipping away.
- Try to use the same plates and cutlery every time to help the person become familiarized with the items every time at meal time.
- It is recommended to use a matching set for the person suffering from dementia. This way, they will be able to distinguish which plate or which cup is theirs.
- If the person suffering from dementia starts to find it very difficult to use utensils, keep encouraging them to use them. However, start to slowly introduce finger foods into their meals, as they will find it easier to eat those.
- Don't use plastic utensils or Styrofoam cups. Because of their texture, a person with dementia might be tempted to eat them, and this will cause severe issues (it can lead to choking, for example).
- Be ready for unexpected combinations and for the patient to develop new tastes.

Dementia Patients and Sleeping

Sleeping may be normal and natural for healthy people, but for those suffering from dementia, it can become a huge issue, both for the patients themselves and for their families.

A dementia patient who doesn't sleep will make it worse for themselves, as this could worsen their worst behaviors and it might alter their entire mindset. In fact, lack of sleep can be a problem for healthy people as well, and it can worsen their behavior - but when the problems associated with a lack of sleep are overlapped on the problems associated with someone who suffers from Alzheimer's or dementia, things can easily become difficult to manage.

Even more, when a person who suffers from dementia doesn't sleep, those around him/her might not sleep as well, which can increase tension in the household and can worsen the situation, bringing it to an entirely different level of difficulty.

There is no single cause that leads people with dementia to sleep less. Rather, you should look at a collection of common causes and identify which one is right in the case of the person you care for.

Some of the most frequent causes for lack of sleep in dementia include the following:

- Aging. As we grow older, we all tend to sleep less and spend less time in the "deep sleep" phase. This is largely due to the fact that the circadian rhythm itself is altered as we grow older. Since most of the dementia patients discover their disease as they get older, this might be correlated with the aging process itself.
- Chronic conditions and some types of medications can also affect sleep. Sometimes, older adults experience both the sleep trouble that comes with aging and the sleep trouble that comes with certain medical conditions. In these cases, treating these causes might help a person suffering from Alzheimer's or dementia to sleep better. Some of the conditions associated with poor sleep include:
    - Certain conditions related to the heart and the lungs (heart failure, chronic obstructive pulmonary disease, and so on).
    - Certain conditions related to the stomach, like the gastroesophageal reflux disease.
    - Some types of chronic pain (e.g. arthritis)
    - Conditions connected to the urinary system that make older people more prone to waking up at night to urinate (e.g. enlarged prostate, overactive bladder, etc.)
    - Conditions connected to one's mood (e.g. anxiety, depression, and so on).
    - Some types of medications, as well as substance use (such as alcohol, for example)
- Underlying sleep disorders worsen as we get older. If someone suffered from a sleep related breathing disorder (such as sleep apnea), the condition might get worse as the person is getting older.
- The nature of Alzheimer's (as well as that of other neurodegenerative diseases) affects the way we sleep. When the brain is deteriorated (such as in the case of Alzheimer's, for example), this might affect the way the brain functions at night. As a consequence, people suffering from Alzheimer's might have more awake time. In other types of dementia (such as Lewy Body or Parkinson's Disease, for example), REM sleep behavior disorder may appear. This disorder causes the patient to experience very swift, almost violent movements during their sleep.

Sometimes, these symptoms can be noticeable before any of the other major symptoms experienced in this type of dementia.

Most of us will sleep lighter and less as we age. However, seniors who suffer from dementia or Alzheimer's in particular might be more affected by these natural processes as they grow older and as their illness progresses. This is why it is of the utmost importance for you as a caretaker to make sure your loved one sleeps well at night.

While you might not be able to control the actual sleep quality, pattern, or time, there are things you can do to make the situation better. Some of the very best situations here include the following:

- Spending time outdoors or in rooms filled with natural light during the day. This helps the body stay on track with its circadian signals (the signals that help us live around the 24-hour day). If the person cannot get outside for at least one hour every day, you might want to consider investing in a bright light therapy lamp.

- Physical activity during daytime. Walking can help the sleep quality, and it is the kind of physical exercise people with Alzheimer's can take.

- Create a sleep routine that triggers the patient to want to sleep. For instance, when sleeping time comes, you might want to make the sleeping environment darker and quieter. This should be maintained throughout the entire night.

- The wake up time should be included in the routine as well. Ideally, the person suffering from dementia should go to sleep and wake up at around the same times every day.

- Sleep medication can be administered for patients with dementia as well. However, before you get to that, first check the current medication the person is taking and whether or not this type of drug is affecting their sleep. This is quite the plausible scenario, since some sedating medications administered during daytime might cause the patient to sleep too much during the day (and thus, make them unable to sleep at night).

When this is not a root cause, you might want to consider offering the patient medication. However, it is extremely important that sleep medication should be the last option. Sleeping pills, sedatives, benzodiazepines, and even over the counter sleep helpers can improve the patient's sleep quality.

Yet, the fact that more pills have to be added to the daily routine and the fact that some of these medications are very dangerous when taken in larger amounts than recommended make them the last option for people who suffer from dementia.

Even more, the vast majority of the sleeping medication out there can cause severe side effects for those who suffer from dementia. In some cases, they worsen the levels of cognition. In others, they pose a direct risk of death.

Some of the least dangerous sleep meds that can be administered to patients with Alzheimer's include Melatonin (a hormone normally secreted by the human body to help with the sleep-wake cycle) and Trazodone (a weak antidepressant that causes mild sedation).

Even though these drugs do exist and they might work, it is still recommended to take the natural path as much as you can. If you have done everything in your power to try and improve the sleeping pattern, time, and quality of the person you are caring for and you still cannot see any results, do talk to your doctor about this. A geriatrician will be able to suggest alternatives to help your loved one sleep better and more.

Dementia is the kind of diagnosis that may come like a strike of lightning. It is usually sudden, unexpected, and it leaves permanent scars not only for the person diagnosed with any of the illnesses in the dementia spectrum, but for the loved ones as well.

Dementia should not and must not mean the end of life. Adjustments have to be made and some areas of your life might change entirely. Yet, a sense of wonder, beauty, and happiness can still remain. It is of the utmost importance to stay positive, as the person who was diagnosed and as the person(s) who will take care of the person diagnosed.

The situations described in this chapter are not meant to scare you, but to prepare you for what is to come and to show you that there are solutions that will make life better, even as the disease progresses.

Stay strong!

Chapter 9: Dementia Resources

As I mentioned at the very beginning of this book, dementia is far more commonly known and understood than it used to be. Some people still mistake dementia for Alzheimer's, and "dementia" as a popular term might still be used to describe "crazy" - but these are common misconceptions that are slowly leaving the mainstream landscape.

Fortunately, people diagnosed with dementia, as well as people who surround those who have been diagnosed with this range of disorders, have a lot more resources at hand so that they can manage their situation as well as they can.

Some of the most important resources include the following:

Dementia Friendly America:

https://www.dfamerica.org/resources

BrightFocus Foundation:

https://www.brightfocus.org

The National Institute of Aging:

https://www.nia.nih.gov/

Alzheimer's Association: https://alz.org/professionals/healthcare-professionals/care-planning

Alzheimer's Associations Around the world:

https://www.alz.co.uk/associations

These sites will provide you with a good starting point in learning more about dementia, Alzheimer's disease, and everything they entail. They might not give you all the answers (including the most important one: *why*). But even so, they might help you understand the situation a little better and they might help you find solutions for common issues people living with dementia encounter.

As a caretaker, you should be more than well informed. The life and the quality of life of the person you are taking care of are in your hands. Their emotions are in their own hands many times, but their *present* is in your hands.

I strongly encourage you to read as much as possible and to ask all the questions you may have. As mentioned above, you might not always get the answers, but you can definitely hope that, one day, the unanswered questions will find their path back to you. Research is being done in this field more than in many other fields of medicine - and while we may not be very close to an actual cure, we are discovering new answers every day. They might not change the outcome of such a diagnosis, but they might change the way you perceive it and the way you take action when dealing with it on a daily basis.

If, as a caretaker, you have to quit your job and still support your family, I strongly encourage you to research ways of making money at home as well. With the internet at your fingertips, you have many options when it comes to earning a decent living while still being able to attend to your loved one or parent.

You could create handcrafted pieces, you could write, or you could provide simple Virtual Assistant services that will help you maintain your financials on top of the mad situation life has thrown you into. You can learn more about making a living at home from the following sites:

This Scott Alan Turner blog post: https://scottalanturner.com/50-legitimate-ways-to-make-money-from-home-in-2016/

This article from Entrepreneur.com:

https://www.entrepreneur.com/article/306578

The Smart Passive Income Blog by Pat Flynn:

https://www.smartpassiveincome.com/

Upwork, one of the major freelancing platforms in the world:

https://www.upwork.com/

Also as a caretaker, you might want to look into resources that will help you stay positive along the way. It will be difficult, no doubt - but it is not completely impossible. And, in fact, it is essential for the overall success of your entire effort to make a patient's life better.

Some of the sites you might want to visit for this include:

The Positive Psychology Program:

https://positivepsychologyprogram.com

Happier Human:

https://www.happierhuman.com

Positivity Strategist:

http://positivitystrategist.com

Furthermore, it is important for you stay in touch with people who are going through the same difficulties as you are. Search for support groups in your area, connect with people online who are also caretakers for people living with dementia, and don't hesitate to search for stories online that will help you feel more in touch with the hardships of dealing with such a disease.

Conclusion

Dementia must not be taken as the end of a journey. It is a disease that can severely affect your life and the lives of those around you, and it is a disease that drastically lowers the life expectancy - but, depending on when the diagnosis is made, it can mean that you still have many years ahead of you.

Yes, nobody can lie to you: dementia will affect every area of your life in ways you did not perceive before this diagnosis came into your life like a meteor, out of nowhere, with no apparent signs. From the way your house is arranged to your daily habits and to the things you can do with your loved one or parent, everything will change. At first, changes will be minor - but since this is a progressive, degenerative disease, you can expect things to get worse.

Dementia is, by and large, one of the most cruel illnesses mankind has ever known. Not only does it steal your physical abilities, but it steals one of the single most important treasures a human being can hold in the later stage of their life: their memories. The more you forget, the less *you* you will feel. And the more of yourself you lose, the more you will feel withdrawn and depressed.

Dementia comes with a snowball effect: at first, it is the minor slippages, the things you forget, the slight motor skill loss, the pain and aches you may even dismiss as pure signs of aging. As the illness progresses, though, you will find that dementia is ready to take everything away from you, like a thief that is too greedy and too willing to hurt.

As the person standing by someone who is diagnosed with dementia, you will feel robbed of everything you have built for the past years and decades. You will feel that someone entered your house, took over, and stole the most precious and beautiful thing you ever had: your relationship with your loved one or parent.

Dementia is not like other diseases threatening to steal the person you love. It steals bits and pieces of them until nearly nothing is left.

Yes, dementia can be a gloomy diagnosis and it can seal your next years in ways you didn't imagine were possible when you said "I do" in front of the altar or when your dad proudly took a photo of you on your high school graduation day. In some cases, the diagnosis can come so early in life that it is nearly impossible to comprehend *what* is going on - or *why* all of this is happening.

Unfortunately, not even modern medicine can answer those questions in full. Research is being done and new results shed light every day - so there is optimism.

Beyond statistical data and promises of cures, you should find your positivity in *yourself*. This is the single most important lighthouse to look after in the journey ahead of you.

This book was not meant to terrify you - it was meant to show you dementia as it is, with its greedy appearance that takes your own stories away from you and your loved ones. There is no point in sugarcoating a diagnosis like this: it is what it is, and this is the first thing you must accept if you want the years left to be spent in as much joy and beauty as possible.

This book was meant to be an introduction into dementia, from what it is to what causes it and how it can be avoided. A journey into discovering that, despite the dark outcome of such a diagnosis, you can still afford to live a good life.

There is hope after dementia. It might not feel like it when vital abilities are stolen from you or your loved ones, but it is in love and kindness that you will eventually find your balance through the harsh times ahead.

Before you change the dining room and make a very clear schedule of what everyday should look like for the person living with dementia, you should first change your mindset as a caretaker. You are there as the support of a person who loved you unconditionally throughout their entire life. You are there to shed light in days when only darkness will hover over their memories and sense of self. You are there to be the one who helps the person diagnosed with dementia to keep on living as beautifully as they can.

Dementia steals a lot of things from you - but what it will never steal is your kindness and your experiences. As the caretaker, you will always have the memories of the years past - and it is your duty to help your loved one or parent to remember the most beautiful moments from before the diagnosis. It is your duty to help them see the light through the clouds of memories that overlap and thoughts that make sense no more. It is your duty to be *there*, heart and soul.

Given the implications of living with someone who has dementia, it can be difficult to asses just how much your life will change - but expecting the worst and preparing for it will help you strengthen your core and be the rock your loved one needs when everything crumbles into pieces.

As someone diagnosed with dementia, it is perfectly understandable why you might not want to share the news with your loved ones. Sooner or later, however, they will have to find out - and it’s always best that they hear it from you and start preparing as soon as possible. Your disease will slowly degenerate and at some point, you might need help for the most basic necessities of living. You *can* choose to go away to a care home and give yourself into the hands of trained staff - but even so, your family and friends should still know about your diagnosis so that they can support you emotionally every time they visit.

It's hard to understand dementia if you have never looked it in the eye, if you have never seen the clouds behind a patient's lost look, or if you have never seen someone degrade so much that they cannot even recognize themselves.

It is hard to understand why things like these are happening to *you* as well. More often than not, dementia comes into people's lives unannounced, without any kind of trigger. Medical science still has a lot of research to do in this respect before we can nail down a very specific reason (or set of reasons) why dementia happens.

The harshest truth of them all is that there is nothing you can do, other than try to live a balanced life from hereon. Sadly, it is a truth you must accept, because there is simply no other truth.

Everything that was described in this book, from the therapies frequently associated with dementia to the very essence of what every day will look like, is meant to help you on the road ahead. The information I have gathered here is meant to make life a little easier, a little happier, and to allow people who have been diagnosed with dementia to live their last years as dignified as they can.

Yes, dementia is incurable.

And yes, most of the time, dementia is the underlying cause of death for a lot of those who are diagnosed with this disorder.

But no, dementia does not have to mean you will lose everything. You can still have candid moments of smiling and laughing with the ones you love. On good days, they might remember sweet moments of your first wedding years or from when you were a toddler and they were helping you walk for the first time. On bad days, things will not be great - but you will always have the memories to look back to, you will always have the support of trained professionals who know how to help people with dementia and their families, and you will always have things you can do to make everything better - even if just for a little bit.

More than anything, I encourage you to stay stronger than ever. The years ahead of you - as a patient or as a caretaker - are anything but easy.

As a caretaker, you are the only strength you have, at the end of the day. You are the only one who can help the patient remember important things when the disease degenerates to a point where every aspect of life is affected. You are the one who will put the spoon in their hand when they forget how to do it. You are the one who will remind them that you are their spouse, their son, or their daughter. You are the one who will be able to put smile on your loved one's face when days are gloomy and everything is shadowed.

As someone suffering from dementia, you must keep your core strong as well. Many people postpone the degeneration of their symptoms for years and live happily together with their families, taking part in some of their most important events: their children's weddings, seeing their first grandsons and granddaughters born, and even seeing them walk and laugh and talk for the first time.

Dementia is cruel - it is as cruel as it gets. It is the kind of diagnosis that might leave you without hope or perspective, and, as a patient, it is a disease that will leave you with nothing but the *present.*

Regardless of whether you are diagnosed with Alzheimer's or other types of dementia, your life will change. But the right outside help and the right mindset can determine just to what extent this change will come in and affect your own situation.

And while dementia is a thief that can leave you with next to nothing in terms of cognitive abilities, it is also a thief that knows not to take away smiles, beauty, the chance to enjoy a flower or a nice perfume, the happiness of a tasty meal or the sporadic memory of a childhood friend who made you laugh.

It is a thief that cannot steal your own strength from you.

A thief you can delay and prepare for.

A thief that can never steal your love. Your love of beauty and grace, your love of the ones who love you, and your love of the present moment.

There are harsh times ahead, and I want to emphasize that it will not be easy for anyone involved. But staying strong and positive are the main things you should cling onto - because, as said above, they are the only guiding lights in these times of sadness and pain.

Thank you for having taken the time to read this - I genuinely believe the information here will prove helpful in preparing you for what lies ahead.

I hope this book will help you build yourself up stronger for what is to come. And I truly hope that the months and years ahead of you will be gentle on you, no matter the way it all turns out in the end!

References

Alzheimer' s Disease Questions and Answers. (2019). Retrieved from https://dshs.texas.gov/alzheimers/qanda.shtm

Creutzfeldt-Jakob Disease Fact Sheet | National Institute of Neurological Disorders and Stroke. (2019). Retrieved from https://www.ninds.nih.gov/Disorders/Patient-Caregiver-Education/Fact-Sheets/Creutzfeldt-Jakob-Disease-Fact-Sheet

Dementia: Incidence and Prevalence. (2019). Retrieved from https://www.asha.org/PRPSpecificTopic.aspx?folderid=8589935289§ion=Incidence_and_Prevalence

Lewy Body Dementia. (2019). Retrieved from https://www.alz.org/alzheimers-dementia/what-is-dementia/types-of-dementia/lewy-body-dementia

Matthews, K. (2019). Retrieved from https://www.alzheimersanddementia.com/article/S1552-5260(18)33252-7/abstract

Memory Vs. Experience: Happiness is Relative. (2019). Retrieved from https://www.psychologicalscience.org/observer/memory-vs-experience-happiness-is-relative

Memory Vs. Experience: Happiness is Relative. (2019). Retrieved from https://www.psychologicalscience.org/observer/memory-vs-experience-happiness-is-relative

Reference, G. (2019). Huntington disease. Retrieved from https://ghr.nlm.nih.gov/condition/huntington-disease

What is FTD?. (2019). Retrieved from https://www.theaftd.org/what-is-ftd/disease-overview/

www.ingramcontent.com/pod-product-compliance
Ingram Content Group UK Ltd.
Pitfield, Milton Keynes, MK11 3LW, UK
UKHW061706190726
13853UKWH00008B/2430